A GUIDE TO LIVING WITH MVP FOR
YOU AND YOUR FAMILY

Coping with Mitral Valve Prolapse

A GUIDE TO LIVING WITH MVP FOR
YOU AND YOUR FAMILY

Coping with Mitral Valve Prolapse

ROBERT H. PHILLIPS, Ph.D.

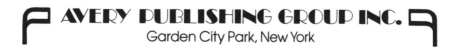
AVERY PUBLISHING GROUP INC.
Garden City Park, New York

The medical information and procedures contained in this book are not intended as a substitute for consulting your physician. All matters regarding your physical health should be supervised by a medical professional.

Cover designers: Rudy Shur and Martin Hochburg
In-house editor: Bonnie Freid
Typesetting: Bonnie Freid

Library of Congress Cataloging-in-Publication Data

Phillips, Robert H., 1948-
    Coping with mitral valve prolapse : a guide to living with MVP for
you and your family / by Robert H. Phillips.
        p. cm.
    Includes bibliographical references and index.
    ISBN 0-89529-514-8
    1. Mitral valve--Displacement--Psychological aspects. I. Title.
RC685.V2P56 1992
616.1'25--dc20   91-46165
                                                          CIP

Copyright © 1992 by Robert H. Phillips, Ph.D.

Printed in the United States of America

10 9 8 7 6 5 4

Contents

Dedication

This book is lovingly dedicated to the special people in my life: my wife, Sharon, and my three sons, Michael, Larry, and Steven; my parents, sister, and grandparents; all my other relatives and in-laws; and my friends.

Acknowledgments

Appreciative words of thanks must be accorded some very special people who provided invaluable assistance in the preparation of this book. Thanks to Ted Webb for critical review, helpful suggestions, and belief in this project. Thanks to Robert Goldstein, M.D., Alan Binder, M.D., Mark Kessler, M.D., and Harlan Krumholz, M.D. for their knowledgeable and helpful reviews of the manuscript. And thanks to Michele Walsh, Ann Dominger, and Larry Phillips for the hours spent transcribing, revising, and typing the manuscript.

Foreword

The mitral valve prolapse syndrome of chest pain, panic attacks, anxiety, and fatigue has been controversial since it was first described. There has been considerable disagreement about whether the syndrome exists at all. As a result, many patients have been confused about this common heart condition.

Mitral valve prolapse is a medical term that describes an abnormal movement of the mitral valve as the heart beats. Over the past decade, with improvements in our ability to view the heart, the medical community has refined its ability to detect the abnormal movement of the mitral valve known as mitral valve prolapse. We have learned that the condition is extremely common, being present in perhaps 5 percent of the population. Fortunately, it is rare that this abnormality interferes with the efficient pumping of blood by the heart.

Most physicians consider the condition of little consequence, and, for most people, mitral valve prolapse is silent. Many people with mitral valve prolapse, nevertheless, have a variety of bothersome, often very uncomfortable symptoms. Whether the mitral valve abnormality of the heart is directly responsible for the cluster of symptoms including fatigue, chest pain, and panic attacks that constitutes the mitral valve prolapse syndrome is not known. What is not controversial is that many patients with mitral valve prolapse suffer from many symptoms, perceive that their life is less full than it could be, and attribute these feelings to mitral valve prolapse. For these people, learning to cope with mitral valve prolapse is an important challenge.

This book is the perfect remedy for these concerns. Until now, there has been a dearth of good books for the layperson on mitral valve prolapse. There has been a great need for a book that would present a balanced view of the information available on mitral valve prolapse, and would help people cope with their anxiety. There has been a great need for this book!

Dr. Robert Phillips has helped countless people with his books on coping with a variety of chronic conditions, including rheumatoid arthritis and systemic lupus erythematosus. Now, fortunately for people with mitral valve prolapse, he has turned his considerable talents to one of the most prevalent cardiac abnormalities. This book is both easy to read and informative. Best of all, Dr. Phillips defuses many of the common concerns about mitral valve prolapse and helps the reader take charge of the situation. He identifies potential problems and puts forth practical suggestions for coping with them.

I look forward to using this book to help my patients who are troubled by mitral valve prolapse. If you or someone close to you feels that his or her lifestyle has been impaired by mitral valve prolapse, the best treatment may be a prescription for this book.

Harlan M. Krumholz, M.D.
Cardiovascular Division
Beth Israel Hospital
Harvard Medical School
Boston, MA

Preface

Millions of people have mitral valve prolapse. Of these, a smaller percentage experience noticeable physical symptoms. If you're in that category, mitral valve prolapse can have a major impact on you and your family.

You may have many questions about mitral valve prolapse. Some of them can be answered by physicians or other professionals. Others may be answered by the relatively few books or articles on the subject. However, many questions cannot be answered. Why? Scientists just don't know all the answers. This can be upsetting. Also upsetting is the feeling you may experience because you're dealing with a "defect in your heart." You may feel that you're alone because no one understands. Knowing that you have a chronic medical problem can be depressing.

Heavy stuff? You bet it is! But it shows why this book was written. "Why?" you're dying to know. This book, chock-full of information, suggestions, and techniques, was written to help you, the members of your family, and your friends learn how to cope with mitral valve prolapse.

The first part of the book presents basic information about mitral valve prolapse: what it is, what the symptoms are, an overview of treatment techniques, and so on. The other sections deal with different aspects of living with the condition, including coping with emotions, changes in lifestyle, and living with others. These are all important aspects of coping with this or any other chronic medical problem. We will explore them in detail, and you'll find suggestions and strategies as well as illustrative examples for each component. In fact, a lot of the information you'll read can (and does!) apply to any chronic medical condition. In this book, however, the main focus is on your life with mitral valve prolapse.

You'll read general information concerning symptoms. Remember, however: Each person with mitral valve prolapse experiences symptoms differently. Similarly, the psychological consequences of having mitral valve prolapse also vary in each person who is diagnosed with the condition. But by reading the information, you'll realize that you're not alone; others experience a lot of what you do. This can be reassuring. Even though a lot of similarities may exist, your own life with mitral valve prolapse—the way it affects you and the way you experience it—will not be exactly the same as anyone else's. You are a unique person. Therefore it will be up to *you* to use the suggestions and strategies in the book to help you cope as well as you possibly can.

Until such time as there is no longer a condition called mitral valve prolapse, you'll have to live with it. I hope this book will help both you and your family do just that, and do it comfortably. Remember: You can *always* improve the quality of your life.

Robert H. Phillips, Ph.D.
Center for Coping
Long Island, NY

PART I
Mitral Valve Prolapse—
An Overview

1

The Heart and Its Function

Marie, a twenty-eight-year-old mother of two, had not been feeling well. She had been experiencing frightening chest pains, and she felt she had less energy than someone twenty-eight years old should have. At times, the discomfort was so severe that she thought she was having a heart attack!

After much procrastination, Marie went to her physician. He gave her a complete physical examination, carefully listened to her heart, and ordered a number of tests. Finally, he sat down at his desk and prepared to discuss his findings with Marie. Marie nervously approached the chair by his desk and sat down. Her husband of eight years sat by her side. The doctor looked at her and wasted no time in telling her, "Marie, you have mitral valve prolapse." Marie's immediate reaction was similar to the immediate reaction of many individuals diagnosed with this condition. Trembling, she looked at the doctor and exclaimed, "What's mitral valve prolapse??"

So, what is mitral valve prolapse? Mitral valve prolapse (commonly abbreviated as MVP) is the most frequently used name for a condition that has also been called the billowing mitral valve leaflet syndrome, prolapsing mitral valve leaflet syndrome, floppy valve syndrome, Barlow's Syndrome, among other names (what would *you* like to call it???). But what is it? In order to really understand MVP, let's begin by discussing the structure and function of the heart, what

the mitral valve is, and the role the mitral valve plays in the circulatory system.

THE STRUCTURE OF THE HEART

The size of the pump we know as the heart is usually not much larger
than your clenched fist. Its weight is usually about one half pound.

The heart is made up of four chambers, the left and right atria (atria
is the plural of atrium), and the left and right ventricles. The atria are the
top chambers, and the ventricles are the bottom chambers. You could
actually think of the heart as being two pumps. Each atrium/ventricle
combination makes up one of the pumps. In other words, the left atrium
and left ventricle form one pump. The right atrium and right ventricle
form the other pump. In each pump, the atrium is the collecting chamber.
This is where the blood enters the heart. Then it is pumped into the
ventricle, where it is pumped out of the heart once again.

The left side of the heart is separated from the right side of the heart
by the septum, a solid, fibrous wall of muscle. The septum is not the
only muscle in the heart. Muscle surrounds the chambers themselves,
and is what works the contracting or pumping mechanism of the
heart.

WHAT DOES THE HEART DO?

The primary purpose of the heart is to pump blood throughout the
body. Why is it so important for the body to receive this blood? Blood
contains oxygen and nutrients. Every cell of the body needs this
oxygen and these nutrients in order to be nourished and healthy. The
blood also provides a way for wastes, the normal by-product of cell
function, to be removed from the nourished cells.

WHAT IS THE PATH OF THE BLOOD?

Let's picture the trip of the blood starting in the left ventricle. From
this chamber, the heart pumps the blood into the aorta, which is the
main artery leaving the heart. The blood flows through the arteries of
the entire body, nourishing the cells and picking up waste products.
Then the blood comes back to the heart through the veins, returning

to the right atrium. The right atrium pumps the blood into the right ventricle, which pumps the blood through the blood vessels to the lungs. The lungs rid the blood of gaseous wastes such as carbon dioxide and oxygenate the blood. The newly oxygenated blood returns to the left atrium, at the top left side of the heart. It's then pumped through the mitral valve into the left ventricle, where it once again is pumped throughout the body to nourish all the body's cells. This process continues as long as you live.

It is estimated that blood travels completely throughout the body, through all the arteries, capillaries (the tiniest blood vessels), and veins, in approximately sixty seconds. It is also estimated that the blood can travel at speeds of up to ten miles an hour! The fastest speeds come when the powerful left ventricle pumps the blood into the aorta.

Want some more trivia? The heart pumps an average of approximately one hundred thousand times per day. During that period of time it pumps more than two thousand gallons of blood throughout the body. Every time the heart pumps, it pumps approximately two and a half ounces of blood into the blood vessels.

HOW DOES THE HEART WORK?

The left and right atria actually prime (prepare) the ventricles for doing their job of pumping the blood out of the heart. The ventricles are very important, because they provide the pumping power to move the blood throughout the body.

The most powerful pumping comes from the left ventricle. Why? It is from here that the blood has to be pumped throughout the entire body. Because the left ventricle is on the left side of your chest, you often feel like your heart is beating on the left side of your chest. (This doesn't mean, though, that your right ventricle is on the right side of your chest. It's actually centrally located, under, or just slightly to the left of, your sternum.)

Because of the strength needed to pump blood throughout the body, the left ventricle is the largest and thickest of the heart's four chambers. The pressure produced by the left ventricle in pumping the blood is what determines your blood pressure.

The right ventricle, in pumping the blood to the lungs, also generates pressure. But normally, the pressure that is generated by the right ventricle is approximately one fourth of that produced by the left ventricle. Because the pressure produced by the right ventricle is so much less than the left ventricle, the walls and muscle mass of the right ventricle are thinner than those of the left ventricle.

It may sound like the heart's job is a simple one, but it is very complex. All parts of the heart must function in a perfectly timed sequence. This is accomplished by having certain specialized heart cells form an "electrical system." This electrical system serves a number of functions. It sends signals to each part of the heart, triggering activity at appropriate times. It makes sure the left atrium and the right atrium properly prime the ventricles so that they will do their jobs on schedule. It makes sure the millions of cells that make up the heart contract together, and at the right time, in order to provide the necessary pressure to pump the blood to all the places it must reach. The electrical system also insures that the heartbeat continues. In fact, the electrical system of the heart is the body's own natural pacemaker, making sure that the heart is pumping properly and attempting to reestablish normal functioning if any problems occur.

The "pacemaker of the heart" is called the sinoatrial node. This tissue is actually muscular tissue. It is tiny, approximately twenty-five millimeters long and three millimeters thick, and it is located in the upper right part of the heart. This node produces the electrical signals that trigger the heart to pump. The signals also determine how fast or slow the muscles of the heart contract.

So what exactly happens? As the blood fills up each atrium, the sinoatrial node (the pacemaker) sends an electrical signal. This triggers the atrium to contract and pump the blood into the ventricle. The left and right atria pump the blood at approximately the same time. This primes the ventricles. The ventricles receive an electrical impulse a fraction of a second after the top chambers do. This causes the ventricles to pump a fraction of a second after the atria. Remember, all four chambers cannot beat at once because the blood has to flow from one chamber to another in correct sequence in order to work effectively.

WHERE DO THE VALVES COME IN?

Because the blood pumps through and out of the heart as a result of contractions of the chambers, it is essential that the blood pumps only in the correct direction. This is one of the most important requirements of heart function. What makes sure that the blood in the heart continues to flow in the right direction? The valves! These are the flaps that separate each of the chambers. At appropriately triggered times, they open to allow the blood to pump through. Then they close to prevent the blood from flowing back.

There are four main valves in the heart. Two valves separate the atria from the ventricles, and the other two valves separate the ventricles from the blood vessels to which blood is pumped from the ventricles.

To learn the names of each of the valves, let's again consider the flow of the blood. Starting in the left ventricle, the blood is pumped through the aortic valve into the aorta and then to all parts of the body. When it returns to the right atrium, it is pumped through the tricuspid valve into the right ventricle. Then it goes through the pulmonary valve into the blood vessel taking it to the lungs. It returns to the left atrium, where it is pumped through the mitral valve into the left ventricle.

ONE-WAY CONTROL

Both the mitral valve and the tricuspid valve open to allow a free flow of blood from the atria to the ventricles. But even more importantly, they then tightly close to prevent blood from flowing back into the atria when the ventricles contract. The aortic and pulmonary valves open to allow the blood to flow into the main blood vessels leaving the heart, but when the pumping stops they also close tightly to prevent any back flow. So the valves are really working as a one-way control system. This is necessary for good blood circulation.

The valve separating the right ventricle and atrium, the tricuspid valve, has three leaflets or flaps. The valve between the left atrium and ventricle, the mitral valve, has two leaflets.

PROBLEMS WITH THE VALVES

Valves that don't work properly are among the more common heart problems. The mitral valve is the valve that is most vulnerable to damage. If the heart valves are damaged, the leaflets may be unable to close tightly enough to prevent blood backflow. When a valve is unable to close properly and tightly, some of the blood that has already been pumped through it can leak back. This is called regurgitation. If this happens, the chamber that was supposed to have been emptied as a result of the pumping or contraction of the heart partially refills with blood that was just there. This may cause a backup of blood. That's where the name blood regurgitation comes from.

If this happens, the power of the contraction does not just pump the blood in the right direction, but also pumps it backwards. When the valve is not working properly and there is blood regurgitation, the heart has to work harder. Over a period of time, this extra effort can damage the heart. But keep in mind that the heart does have a "reserve capacity"—it does have the ability to handle mild to moderate mitral regurgitation without significant difficulty.

This book focuses on the condition known as mitral valve prolapse. Let's talk about the MVP in more detail.

2

What Is Mitral Valve Prolapse?

In people who have normal mitral valves, when the ventricles of the heart contract, the mitral valve remains firmly and tightly closed. As a result, no blood leaks back into the upper chamber of the heart. (Right! There is no blood regurgitation. See, you're learning the lingo!)

In a person who has MVP, the mitral valve leaflets may not close tightly and properly. One or both of the mitral leaflets bend or snap back into the left atrium during the contraction of the left ventricle. This is where the word prolapse comes from (or the word billow). Prolapse is the term used for the way the valve would flap back into the left atrium after the contraction of the ventricle.

WHY DOES THE VALVE PROLAPSE?

In mitral valve prolapse, there is a defect in the normal structure of the valve's connective tissue. This connective tissue is actually the "backbone" of the valve. When there are problems with this tissue, the leaflets of the valve may become stretched out of shape or get longer. This problem can affect either or both of the leaflets. The leaflet's elongation and loss of strength are why the valve billows or flaps back into the atrium during the ventricle's contraction. This may be due to the shape of the mitral valve, or because of a problem with the connective tissue, or with the little tendons, the cordae, which normally hold the flaps in place.

So MVP is a problem with the anatomy or structure of the valve. If the structure of the valve is defective, the function of the valve changes.

WHO GETS MITRAL VALVE PROLAPSE?

What is known about who gets mitral valve prolapse? In the United States, MVP is the most common heart valve disorder. It is estimated that up to 10 percent (if not more) of the people in the United States have problems with their hearts' mitral valves. This means millions of Americans have MVP. Of course, many of the people who have a mitral valve "abnormality" may never even be aware of it, and therefore may never be diagnosed with MVP. This makes it harder to pinpoint the specific numbers, because there are probably a lot of people who have MVP but have never been actually diagnosed with it.

It seems as though the number of people being diagnosed with MVP is increasing. This is partly because people are more health conscious, and are seeing their doctors more often. It's also because doctors are better able to identify mitral valve prolapse. There has been much improvement in diagnostic testing and there is more awareness of the condition.

MVP Prevalence in Specific Groups

Mitral valve prolapse can occur in all races and ethnic groups. MVP seems to be diagnosed in women almost twice as frequently as men. However, research has suggested that this may, in part, be the result of sociocultural variables, namely, that men are "expected" to be more stoic, less likely to complain, and therefore less likely to present to doctors any MVP symptoms!

What About Age?

The largest percentage of people who are diagnosed with MVP develop the condition and notice it anywhere from the late twenties through the thirties. Although MVP occurs more often in young adulthood, it can occur any time from childhood through the later years.

MVP in Children

MVP occurs in approximately 5 percent of all children. It is probably the most common cardiac diagnosis made in children. As opposed to adults, where women are diagnosed about twice as often as men, boys and girls seem to be diagnosed with MVP in approximately equal numbers.

MVP in Senior Citizens

Some people are diagnosed with MVP in later years, although the numbers are smaller than those diagnosed in young adulthood. An interesting fact is that the number of older men and women diagnosed with MVP are more equal than are younger men and women.

WHAT CAUSES MITRAL VALVE PROLAPSE?

Why does mitral valve prolapse occur? Why do some people experience more symptoms than others? Why, why, why? Researchers continue to try to come up with better answers to these questions.

There can be a number of reasons for problems with the mitral valve, although the exact cause of mitral valve prolapse is still not clearly understood. It is suggested that the possible causes of MVP can be divided into two categories.

Category One: Primary Causes

The first category contains the primary causes. The structural problem of MVP may have been genetically transmitted. It may also have resulted from a congenital birth problem. Mitral valve problems may also result from defects in the tendons controlling the flaps of the valve. Or the flaps may stretch with no apparent cause and without any valve deformity, and just may not close properly. These are examples of primary causes.

Is MVP inherited? One of the few things about MVP that seems to be consistently agreed upon is that the condition is genetically transmitted. The shape of the mitral valve and problems with it are usually hereditary, and can appear in a number of members of the same family. MVP is a dominant condition, but it doesn't develop in every child. However, because of this tendency, if you have MVP, everyone in your immediate family should probably be examined (although it doesn't have to be done today!).

Category Two: Secondary Causes

The second category contains secondary causes. This refers to other diseases and conditions where a malformation of the mitral valve or mitral regurgitation may be a consequence of the primary medical problem. There are many other diseases or conditions that may be associated with MVP. Although many associations have been made between MVP and other diseases, a clear causal relationship has never been determined.

WHAT TRIGGERS MVP?

Many people who have MVP were born with it. There may have always been a problem with the valve, or it may have developed as the person got older. But many people report that, at a specific time, MVP symptoms just "showed up." In many cases, there was some kind of trigger. This trigger could have been either physical or psychological. It could have been a physical stressor, such as an illness or injury, or a psychological stressor, such as some kind of emotional trauma. When a person perceives some type of stressor, the body reacts physically, in addition to psychologically. This physical response may lead to an imbalance in the autonomic nervous system (although it may be hard to connect these two events). Since the autonomic nervous system may be more vulnerable in an individual who has MVP, this imbalance may lead to symptoms of MVP syndrome. This imbalance and any related symptoms may continue until the person is able to reestablish a balance in autonomic nervous system function.

HOW SERIOUS IS MITRAL VALVE PROLAPSE?

MVP is considered to be a condition, rather than a disease. Any chronic medical condition can be serious. Does this mean that because mitral valve prolapse is a chronic condition, everyone with mitral valve prolapse has a serious case of it? No! Although it is a very common condition, and millions of people have it, only a smaller percentage of these people experiences noticeable MVP-related problems.

The severity of mitral valve prolapse varies along a continuum. At the mildest end are those who have a slight problem with the structure of the mitral valve, and experience virtually no symptoms. A large percentage of those with MVP is at this end of the continuum.

At the other, severe end of the continuum are those whose structural and functional variations are more pronounced. They may have more severe mitral valve problems that result in complications such as severe blood regurgitation, endocarditis, or the formation of clots on the valves. Individuals at this end of the continuum require treatment, because the symptoms may be more pronounced. Surgery may even be necessary to replace or reconstruct the mitral valve. This is very rare (estimates are that barely 2 percent of those with MVP will be at this end of the continuum in the first place, and far fewer will require surgery).

The rest of those with MVP fall in between those two extremes, experiencing occasional symptoms of mild to moderate intensity. The symptoms can be an inconvenience at certain times and may be discomforting at other times. But the condition for any of these individuals is not considered to be life-threatening.

However, that doesn't mean that MVP can just be dismissed. Because some of the symptoms can be frightening or because they are uncomfortable, they may interfere with your normal functioning. The anxiety that comes as a result of these concerns, or the discomfort that exists because of the condition, may interfere with your lifestyle and require coping.

Because of the range of intensity of symptoms experienced by those with MVP, it's hard to estimate how many people experience mild symptoms, moderate, severe, or anywhere on the continuum. The important thing, therefore, is that, if you are reading this book, you are looking to improve your ability to cope with whatever symptoms you've got!

In order to understand how serious your own condition is, you should discuss this carefully with your physician. But remember, the severity of mitral valve prolapse is also markedly affected by how well you take care of yourself. Do you stay out until three o'clock in the morning three or four nights each week? Do you make sure that your reputation as a junk-food junkie is firmly intact? If you're on medication, do you take it when you remember to take it, rather than when you should take it? Do you call your physician only when you receive a notice asking if you have moved to another town? Do you allow yourself to be overwhelmed by all kinds of stressful situations? If you use proper health procedures to take care of yourself, take any medication prescribed on schedule, and keep in close contact with your physician, you can decrease the incidence and intensity of MVP symptoms. It is important to remember that any condition, even a mild one, can become serious if it is not taken care of properly. Results usually are good with proper treatment.

Prognosis

The prognosis for those with MVP is quite good. Of course, the prognosis depends on the severity of MVP, any complications that have occurred, and whether or not MVP is primary or secondary. If MVP is secondary, then the prognosis is also determined by the underlying condition that played a role in the development of the valve problem. Since one can never guarantee the prognosis for any one person, it's more important to learn how to best deal with the condition.

Is Mitral Valve Prolapse Fatal?

The most important thing to remember is that MVP, even at its most severe, is not considered to be a life-threatening condition! Why are so many people with MVP afraid that it is? People are often very frightened about things affecting the heart. Since heart attack is still one of the most common causes of death, any chest pain may make you panic, fearing a sudden heart attack. But research has shown that the pain from MVP is not the same as the chest pain of a heart attack.

If you read the medical literature about MVP, you may get frightened. You may read about something called "sudden death."

There are some medical studies in the literature that suggest that individuals with MVP may have a statistically higher risk of sudden death. Very, very rarely does this occur. And, in general, sudden death does not occur specifically because of MVP, but rather, because there are other problems involved. If it does happen (and remember, it's rare) it is the other problems that usually cause it. More often, sudden death may be as a result of long-term coronary artery disease. This is not the same as MVP. MVP is a valve problem.

Older individuals may be at greater risk regarding sudden death (but it's still rare, unless there are other major complications, like coronary disease). So remember: Although MVP may not be life-threatening, it may be lifestyle threatening! That's the reason for coping!

SYMPTOMS OF MITRAL VALVE PROLAPSE

Mitral valve prolapse is a structural problem. There are a number of symptoms, ranging from mild to severe. The most common indication is called a systolic click. This means that if someone listens to your heart with a stethoscope, a click sound can be heard during the ventricle's contraction (called the systole). This click that is heard is the flap of the valve is billowing or flapping back into the atrium. Another indication also heard through the stethoscope is a soft whooshing sound. This is called a late systolic murmur, which means it usually happens at the end of the contraction, and indicates a leakage of blood back through the valve. (What's that called again? Yes, blood regurgitation.)

Blood regurgitation can range from mild to severe. Progressive mitral regurgitation means that the blood leakage problem is getting worse. Other heart problems, such as atrial fibrillation or congestive heart failure, may be a consequence of progressive or severe mitral regurgitation. That's why treatment is required for this.

THE MITRAL VALVE PROLAPSE "SYNDROME"

Many of the ways that MVP affects people goes beyond the click or regurgitation problems mentioned earlier. These ways involve the autonomic nervous system. Let's discuss the autonomic nervous system and the role it plays in mitral valve prolapse.

The Nervous System and MVP

There are actually two major components of the nervous system: the voluntary nervous system and the involuntary nervous system. The voluntary nervous system includes the actions and activities that a person has the ability to control. Examples of voluntary actions that are under the control of the voluntary nervous system are talking, standing, walking, or acting.

The involuntary nervous system is also known as the autonomic nervous system. Any functions of the body that are not consciously controllable are actually controlled by the involuntary or autonomic nervous system. Examples of these functions include blood vessel contraction and blood pressure, relaxation of the blood vessel contractions, sweating, heart rate, respiration, the balance between sleepfulness and wakefulness, and the contraction and dilation of the pupils of the eyes.

The Role of the Autonomic Nervous System

As you know, the body is made up of many systems, such as the circulatory system, respiratory system, and the excretory system. The autonomic nervous system, to at least some degree, plays a role in the smooth functioning of every one of the body's systems. The effectiveness of the autonomic nervous system depends on a proper balance between its two major components: the sympathetic and the parasympathetic nervous system.

What Do They Do?

The easiest way to remember the functions of these two components of the autonomic nervous system is that, with regard to any system of the body, one component (the sympathetic) of the autonomic nervous system "speeds it up," and the other (the parasympathetic) "slows it down." In other words, they act in opposite directions, resulting in a type of "checks and balances" operation. Because of the balance that exists between these two systems, neither component is ever in complete control. Circumstances determine which one is in more control at a particular moment. For example, stress might cause the sympathetic to speed up the body for "self-protection." After the stress is over, the parasympathetic slows down the system. But the balance of control swings back and forth automatically (that's why it's the autonomic nervous system, right?).

There are times that a slight problem may develop in this balancing act. In other words, the "checks and balances" between the two components of the autonomic nervous system may be out of whack and may affect any of the body's systems. This imbalance in the autonomic nervous system is called dysautonomia.

What happens when there is an imbalance between the sympathetic and the parasympathetic systems? There are a number of different possibilities. For example, maybe the sympathetic nervous system will take over too much control, accelerating the body too much. Or maybe the parasympathetic nervous system is not strong enough, so it is unable to slow down a body system. Maybe the parasympathetic nervous system is too strong and it keeps a body system functioning too slowly, not allowing the sympathetic nervous system to make it productive enough. In some cases, maybe both the parasympathetic and the sympathetic nervous systems can at the same time be too active or too underactive. The way anyone experiences this imbalance can vary, as can the degree of imbalance that exists.

By now, you're probably starting to wonder, "Why does all this matter?" Here's the kicker: It has been found that many of the symptoms that occur in individuals who have MVP may be related to an imbalance of the autonomic nervous system! In MVP, this imbalance is usually mild, although it can cause a number of different symptoms (more about this later).

Why the Connection?

Quite a bit of research has suggested that when there is a slight problem in the structure of the mitral valve, there is also a problem in the development, function, or balance of the components of the autonomic nervous system. Although it still is not completely known for sure, one possible explanation is that the autonomic nervous system is formed at approximately the same time that the mitral valve of the heart is formed.

Research has suggested that six specific symptoms, probably resulting from an autonomic nervous system imbalance, are the most common reasons for individuals (who end up being diagnosed with MVP) to seek treatment. These six common symptoms are fatigue, chest pain, palpitations, headaches, dizziness, and panic. None of these are symptoms that are directly associated with MVP as a structural problem, but, instead, are part of the syndrome that is commonly associated with MVP. So the structural problem of MVP, along with an imbalance in the autonomic nervous system, seems to go hand in hand in what has recently begun to be called Mitral Valve Prolapse Syndrome.

Many health professionals in the past, without really understanding the whole syndrome, have labeled individuals with MVP as neurotic. Why? Well, consider the symptoms! Things such as anxiety and panic attacks, fatigue, palpitations, and unusual chest pain, all of unexplainable origin, all unobservable, made these professionals wonder if the symptoms weren't all in the person's head.

Because it is most likely that many people who have only a mild structural variation of the mitral valve, and don't experience these symptoms may not even decide to read this book, we will use the terms MVP and MVP Syndrome interchangeably from this point on. After all, it's the package you want to cope with, right?

THE HISTORY OF MITRAL VALVE PROLAPSE

Will knowing the history of mitral valve prolapse help you feel better? Probably not, but some people are curious as to where things come from. Read on if you like. You will not be quizzed on names and dates!

MVP syndrome has been around for a long time. Symptoms of mitral valve prolapse had been noticed by physicians for hundreds of years, even though the condition had not yet been given its current name. MVP only really became a specific diagnosed medical syndrome in the early 1960s.

As far back as 1871, it was called Irritable Heart, or Da Costa's Syndrome. The condition became more prevalent during and after World War I. Many soldiers were experiencing a lot of the stress and hardship of war. They complained of experiencing shortness of breath, chest pain, flutters in heartbeat, and extreme fatigue. So, in 1914, it became known as Soldier's Heart, a term that had actually originated at the time of the Civil War. It was also called Effort Syndrome. In 1918, it was called Neurocirculatory Asthenia.

After the World War I was over, more and more women were entering the work force. At the same time they were continuing their domestic responsibilities as wives and mothers. Because of this added stress, they were starting to experience the same symptoms that men with "Soldier's Heart" had been experiencing. However, by 1941, a new label was being used to describe the problem: "anxiety neurosis."

Many years later, in the 1960s, a physician named Barlow noticed that women who had this condition had a noticeable click when a stethoscope was used to listen to the heart. This then became known as Systolic Click Syndrome or Barlow Syndrome, since he was the first person to describe this finding. It was also labeled Systolic Click/Late Systolic Murmur Syndrome. And finally in the 1970s and the 1980s it became known as Mitral Valve Prolapse Syndrome.

SYMPTOMS OF MITRAL VALVE PROLAPSE SYNDROME

What are some of the main symptoms of the MVP syndrome? We've already mentioned the most common symptoms that lead someone to the doctor's office. Let's review some of the main symptoms.

Chest Pain

Some individuals with MVP syndrome have occasional chest pain. These pains usually feel like sharp or stabbing pains. They may last from minutes to hours. Occasionally, the pain may feel like angina pain, which may make the person decide to consult a cardiologist.

Palpitations

Palpitations are another very common symptom. These palpitations may appear as a result of exertion, but they also may appear at rest and even during the night. Tachycardia (rapid heart rate) or arrhythmias (irregular heartbeats) may be two of the main causes of the palpitations.

Fatigue

Fatigue is another common symptom of MVP Syndrome. Fatigue can affect people for many reasons, and is a common symptom of many medical problems in addition to MVP.

Other Symptoms

Shortness of breath is also a common symptom of MVP Syndrome, as is anxiety. In some cases, panic attacks may be associated with MVP.

Other symptoms experienced by some individuals with MVP include a resting heartbeat that may be slightly rapid. The heart may respond inappropriately when the person stands up. How? The heartbeat may accelerate too much or not enough. Blood vessels may respond inappropriately to a stressful or active situation. Lower blood pressure may result if the blood vessels do not constrict properly. Higher blood pressure, or reduced circulation to the extremities, may result from the blood vessels constricting too much. Inappropriate heart rate and blood pressure problems may lead to coldness or numb extremities, especially the hands and feet. These are fairly common MVP complaints.

Other than these common symptoms, there are many other symptoms that people with MVP can experience. Among the other symptoms reported by people with MVP are sleep disorders, irritable bowel syndrome or other intestinal problems, stomach problems, dizziness, headaches, and many others. Of course, nobody experiences all of the symptoms. But any of them can be upsetting and they need to be dealt with while efforts are being made to improve them.

Most children who have MVP do not have all of these symptoms. Some of them, however, do have palpitations or chest pain. Children who do have palpitations or chest pain should have a full evaluation, so that treatment can control these symptoms.

COMPLICATIONS

Yes, it is possible for serious complications to occur in people who have MVP. Fortunately, however, complications are not very common.

Complications that are related to MVP include: infective endocarditis, progressive mitral regurgitation that, in rare cases, may require mitral valve surgery, ruptured cordae tendonae, forming of clots, ventricular arrhythmias, and congestive heart failure.

Infective Endocarditis

Infective endocarditis, an infection of the mitral valve, is also called bacterial endocarditis. Only a small percentage of individuals with MVP develop this problem, so the chances of infective endocarditis occurring with MVP is usually small. Those people who have a murmur that indicates mitral regurgitation are at greater risk of developing endocarditis than those who just have a systolic click. Therefore, monitoring should occur. However, endocarditis can occur in individuals even though they don't have mitral regurgitation.

Progressive Mitral Regurgitation

The person's mitral valve is becoming less and less effective, and more and more blood is returning into the atrium when the ventricle contracts. This has serious consequences for the heart, and for the body in general. Simply not enough blood is circulating through the body, and the heart is working too hard.

Ruptured Cordae Tendonae

This is a more common complication of MVP. If the tendons that control the valve flaps rupture, the effectiveness of the leaflet is significantly reduced. This may lead to even more of a mitral regurgitation problem. However, this does not mean that additional aggressive treatment, such as surgery, is always necessary. Symptoms may still be comparatively minor.

It is still not completely understood how many of the symptoms, or even the complications of MVP Syndrome, are really directly caused by the condition, and how many just seem to be associated with it. Some scientists feel that people who experience infective endocarditis, stroke, or serious arrhythmias, or sudden death, who also have MVP, may be experiencing these things as associated events rather than their being caused by MVP. Endocarditis is probably the one major exception. Clearly, individuals who have mitral regurgitation may experience a growth of bacteria on the mitral valve that can lead to endocarditis.

Fortunately, many of these complications are relatively rare. In general, the complications, as well as how serious they are, increase as the person's age increases. That doesn't mean, however, that everyone with MVP gets worse as they get older. In fact, most people don't!

An interesting fact is that although MVP is much more common in women, endocarditis and major mitral insufficiency (possibly requiring surgery) is more often found in men.

Senior citizens may experience MVP complications as a result of chronic MVP. These complications include severe chest pain, cardiac arrhythmias, formation of emboli in the arteries, or progressive mitral regurgitation that may lead to congestive heart failure. Progressive mitral regurgitation may be more of a problem for seniors than for younger individuals.

3

How Is Mitral Valve Prolapse Diagnosed?

After Marie got over her initial shock at being diagnosed with mitral valve prolapse, she asked her doctor to explain how he finally concluded that she had the condition. He told her about the procedures physicians use in accurately diagnosing MVP.

So what is done? How do physicians determine if someone has mitral valve prolapse?

Diagnosis can be easy if the symptoms "paint a picture" for the diagnosing physician. The diagnosis of mitral valve prolapse is properly made as a result of your medical history, combined with a detailed physical examination, and an assessment of appropriate laboratory test results.

The most important first step in diagnosing MVP is the physical examination. During the physical exam, the doctor listens to your heart with a stethoscope. A unique sound, called a "click," will usually be heard in someone who has MVP. This click occurs when the mitral valve snaps or billows back into the heart's upper chamber when the ventricle contracts.

Doctors also will be listening for a soft murmur that may occur at the end of the contraction. This would mean that there is a slight flow of blood back into the upper chamber (mitral regurgitation), because the mitral valve is not closing tightly. Some (but not all) people with MVP also have this soft murmur. Now you know why MVP is sometimes called the click-murmur condition. The click and murmur information obtained by listening with a stethoscope may be called auscultatory findings. Sometimes, physical exams don't disclose MVP right away. Why? The click or the murmur may only be intermittent, so it might be missed.

If the mitral valve doesn't work properly, this is called mitral insufficiency. Your physician needs to determine how severe the mitral insufficiency is. Because mitral insufficiency makes the left ventricle work harder, the size and the performance of the left ventricle can provide a way of determining how severe the problem is.

So your doctor can suspect MVP by listening to the heart through a stethoscope. But it is usually not sufficient to confirm the diagnosis this way. Even though hearing the systolic click or murmur suggests MVP, doctors will usually confirm the diagnosis with more accurate scientific technology.

THE ECHOCARDIOGRAM

Today, the echocardiogram, which only really became part of medical technology in the 1960s, is the test that is most often used to diagnose MVP. If the doctor notices the click or the murmur, the next step often is a recommendation to go for an echocardiogram. This test is designed to indicate if there are any problems with the structure of your heart.

How does it work? The echocardiogram uses sound waves that "echo" or bounce off the heart's structures, creating the pictures that illustrate the exact anatomy of the heart. The pictures that are formed by the sound waves will show if there are any abnormalities in the structure of the mitral valve. It helps the diagnostician to determine the intactness or prolapse of the mitral valve. MVP can usually be accurately diagnosed as a result of this test.

The nice thing about the echocardiogram is that it is non-invasive. It does not involve penetrating the body with anything (other than soundwaves!). No injections are required and it is painless. Thank goodness!

The echocardiogram also can be useful in determining the presence of infective endocarditis. So it may be used later on in your experience with MVP, not just to confirm a diagnosis.

THE ANGIOGRAM

The angiogram is a procedure that involves injecting a dye through the blood vessels and into the heart, and then analyzing the resulting pictures for structural defects. The angiogram is considered by some professionals to be even more accurate in diagnosing MVP than the echocardiogram. The reason it is not used as much is because it is an invasive procedure (it requires an injection). As a result, only under rare or unusual circumstances will physicians resort to angiograms to diagnose MVP.

DO YOU HAVE MVP SYNDROME?

If a structural problem is found, confirming an MVP diagnosis, the next step is to determine if MVP syndrome exists. Depending on the symptoms you've described, your doctor may now look for clinical evidence of problems with your autonomic nervous system or endocrine systems.

Remember that not everybody who is diagnosed with MVP also will have the symptoms normally associated with MVP syndrome, although quite a large number of people will experience overlap in these two diagnoses.

It is not uncommon for individuals who ultimately are diagnosed with MVP to report that they have been previously incorrectly diagnosed with other conditions. After treatment for other conditions did not alleviate all the symptoms, they may have then proceeded with further evaluation, until MVP may have finally been diagnosed. What other conditions have some people been misdiagnosed with? Among the culprits are hypoglycemia, depression, premenstrual syndrome, thyroid problems, anxiety disorders, and even hyperventilation problems. No wonder MVP can drive people crazy!

4

How Is MVP Treated?

So far, we have discussed many things about MVP, including what it is, who may get it, what some of the symptoms are, and how it may be diagnosed. Terrific, but now what you'll really want to know is how you can feel better. True?

You probably have some important questions. What will your doctors do? What will doctors tell you to do? What is the treatment for mitral valve prolapse and how will it affect you? How do you control your symptoms? How do you help yourself get back into the mainstream of life? Let's begin to answer some of the questions about the treatment of mitral valve prolapse.

YOUR ROLE IN TREATMENT

There are always things you can do to help yourself. It doesn't matter how much medical knowledge you have. There are also things you can do that will make your condition worse, but obviously those are things to be avoided. To start helping yourself, you'll want to identify those things that improve your condition and those things that hurt it.

Physicians can provide much in the way of medical information, medication, and expertise. Family and friends can provide emotional support, caring, and guidance. But you are the only one who can make the many small decisions necessary to organize your lifestyle as effectively as possible. These decisions may be small, but they may be critical in determining how MVP affects you. Therefore, it is obvious that you can play an important role in influencing the way you feel. But that's not enough. No single factor is enough. To help yourself best, a whole package approach is essential, where you help yourself in as many ways as possible, both medically and psychologically.

WHAT IS THE GOAL OF TREATMENT?

The goal of treatment is to do the best possible job to keep your health intact, and to minimize any problems that MVP might cause. Treatment for MVP is usually conservative when the only symptoms experienced are those such as chest pain, fatigue, or palpitations. It may be that only education, reassurance, and coping strategies are necessary.

Part of the goal of treatment is to strengthen your body. You'll want to reduce the impact of any symptoms that do occur. Remember that many people with MVP have few or no symptoms. If you do have only minor manifestations of MVP, you'll probably only need to be reassured that you'll be fine, and you'll want to be aware of what you may need to do to prevent infective endocarditis. But if you do experience some symptoms of MVP, the goal of your treatment will be to reduce both the symptoms themselves, and any impact that they may have on your life.

WHAT ARE THE COMPONENTS OF TREATMENT PROGRAMS?

According to many professionals, the most important component in treatment programs for MVP is successful coping—learning to have a positive mental attitude. Having a positive mental attitude will certainly be one of the most important stabilizing forces. In some cases, this, along with reassurance from doctors, may be all that is necessary to live comfortably with MVP.

There are many practical things that can be done to help to improve your mental attitude. We will be talking about many of them in subsequent chapters in the book.

In addition to having a positive mental attitude, there are a number of other things that are important parts of treatment regimens for MVP. Stress management, exercise, proper nutrition and dietary control, and medication where appropriate, are all very important components.

Stress Management

Stress management is a very important part of treatment for MVP. Stress management includes a number of different strategies, dealing with both physiological and psychological stress. An important goal in stress management is to improve your feeling of being in control both of feelings and behaviors.

Exercise

Exercise is also an important part of treatment. Exercise can help you feel better physically, as well as reduce stress and improve your self-esteem. It can also be very helpful in improving the way you perceive your health.

Although some people with MVP may have been told to avoid physical exertion, it has been repeatedly found that a gradually increasing program of physical exercise can be helpful if you have MVP. It can improve muscle tone and stabilize heartbeat. It can improve cardiac function and reduce MVP symptoms. Of course, any exercise should only be done under strict medical supervision.

Nutrition

Dietary modifications and proper nutrition are important because they help to maintain the best possible balance of the autonomic nervous system. For some individuals, intake of sugar and caffeine, or chemicals that inappropriately stimulate the autonomic nervous system, such as caffeine, alcohol, tobacco, or other drugs, should be reduced, if not eliminated.

Drinking plenty of fluids also may be an important part of the treatment program. Fluid intake is important because blood pressure relates to proper intake of fluid. In addition, if blood pressure can be stabilized, this can help to reduce some of the unpleasant symptoms of MVP.

Medical Components of Treatment

If symptoms continue despite other treatment components, medication may be appropriate. One of the problems with using medication, of course, is that it doesn't always alleviate all of the symptoms. And you also may have to deal with the possibility of side effects.

In more severe long-term cases, surgery may be suggested. Surgery is usually only considered if it is necessary to correct severe mitral regurgitation. Surgery using valve replacement can be effective. But, if possible, reconstructive surgery of the valve is preferred.

Other Considerations

It is important that people with MVP not overexert themselves. And, they also should reduce any potential interfering factors or strain on the circulatory system such as being overweight or being anemic. Smoking, as a habit, should be kicked!

EACH PERSON WITH MVP IS UNIQUE

Your experience with mitral valve prolapse is unique. As a result, your physician will set up a treatment program based specifically on your needs.

Because there is no absolute treatment, modifications may be necessary before your treatment program works best. Does that mean that no physicians agree on how mitral valve prolapse should be treated? No. There is a lot of agreement. Most physicians do prescribe similar treatment programs for their patients, depending on the severity of their symptoms, but yours will be adjusted appropriately for you as an individual.

It is very important for you to feel at ease with your physician. You want to have confidence in the treatment program prescribed for you. Imagine this: You hear of somebody else with MVP receiving different treatment from a different physician. You start to believe that the other treatment program might be better. You start losing confidence in your treatment plan, and then in your own physician. Not a great feeling, is it? Remember, there is no one answer! What works for somebody else will not necessarily work for you.

Remember that regardless of the support that you have from the people around you, including family, friends, and professionals, you are the person who is ultimately responsible for doing the best you can to take care of yourself. You are the person who can make the necessary changes, work to improve your positive attitude, and deal as productively as you can with the condition.

TO SUMMARIZE . . .

Professionals involved with the treatment of MVP recognize that the best, most effective treatment program incorporates five major components: (1) adjustment of general lifestyle, involving changes in behavior and activity necessitated by your condition; (2) coping with emotional reactions, because it is so important that stress and negative emotions be controlled, and that you have a positive mental attitude; (3) attention to diet and nutritional needs; (4) exercise, to keep your stamina high; and (5) proper medication, or other medical intervention, when necessary. Each of these components will be discussed in detail in subsequent chapters. But isn't it great to know that there are always things that you can do to improve the way you live and deal with your condition?

PART II
Your Emotions

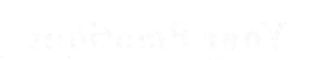

5

Coping With
Your Emotions—
An Introduction

How do you feel about having mitral valve prolapse? (What a question!) Well, each person's emotional responses to MVP is different. Even your own reactions to the condition will vary from time to time. The more severe your reactions are, the more they will interfere with your ability to cope.

Your emotions can ride the roller coaster, just like the way you feel with MVP can vary. As a matter of fact, emotional ups and downs are very common. One of the most important ingredients in successfully living with MVP is to be able to be in control of your emotions.

Your emotional reactions to mitral valve prolapse may start even before treatment has begun. Of course, your reaction will also depend on how suddenly your condition developed. For example if, without any warning symptoms, you were suddenly diagnosed with MVP, you might not adjust as well as if you had been experiencing symptoms for a while.

This is one of the reasons that it is so important to have a positive mental attitude. Individuals with positive mental attitudes can be much more able to be in control of their emotions. So this is a primary goal. Having a negative mental attitude may exacerbate any of the emotional problems that may occur because of, or in addition to, MVP. Therefore one of the first priorities may be to see what you can do to improve your attitude in order to help every other aspect of your functioning as well.

FACTORS SHAPING YOUR EMOTIONAL REACTIONS

A number of factors may play a role in determining how you react to mitral valve prolapse. Keep in mind, however, that because there are so many factors, no one can predict how any person will react at any given time.

How did you handle problems before your condition was diagnosed? What was your general coping style? Were you calm or nervous? Were you persistent or did you give up easily? The way you handle life's problems in general will indicate how well you will cope with mitral valve prolapse and its treatment.

Your age has a bearing on how you respond emotionally. Your general physical health prior to the onset of MVP also plays a role in determining your coping ability. What about your relationships? In many cases, your emotional reactions may reflect the responses of significant people in your life. For example, if family members or friends are anxious about your medical condition, this may affect your emotional reactions.

WHAT EMOTIONAL PROBLEMS?

Have you felt intense anger because you have to go through all this? Are you angry that your life may change because of MVP? Are you afraid of a problem that involves your heart? Are you afraid of the medication you may need? Do you become depressed when you compare your present life to the way things were? Have you felt afraid of not being able to cope? Some of the more common emotional reactions to MVP are depression, fear, anger, and guilt. Because of the importance of coping with these emotions, a separate chapter has been devoted to each of them. But other than these specific emotional responses, what else might you experience?

Do you like yourself less since your diagnosis? Previous feelings of confidence can be quickly shattered. This loss of self-esteem can have a very unpleasant effect on you. You may not feel or behave like yourself. You'll want to deal with this right away in order to return to effective, efficient functioning.

You may feel disoriented. Do you sometimes feel that things around you are unreal? One of the most frightening feelings is that you're not yourself, especially if you don't know why you're feeling this way. It can be reassuring to understand that this happens for many people from time to time. And it can go away.

How about mood swings? Do you ever experience these? Many individuals with MVP do. You may be concerned that this is just because of the syndrome. But if you stop to think about it, everyone experiences mood swings from time to time, whether they have MVP or not! It is possible that certain medications may even increase the range of these mood swings. But let your physician know what's going on, so changes can be made.

MANAGING EMOTIONAL REACTIONS

Some of the ways people have adjusted to MVP and its treatment have included education, support groups, and even therapy, where necessary. Because your emotions play such an important role in life with MVP, you'll certainly want to do the best possible job controlling them. How? Let's discuss some of the more important ways.

Information Gathering

Books may be able to help you generate a more positive mental attitude. There are so many books in the library and in bookstores that offer suggestions for improving one's attitude that it would certainly be a good idea to look into some of them. If you get simply one good idea out of a 300-page book, it makes the reading of the entire book worthwhile. Remember, this is your life we're talking about. You want to do whatever you can to maximize the positive aspects of your life. And improving your attitude is a very important component of that.

Support Groups

Self-help or support groups can be very helpful. You'll see how others handle problems, some of which may be the same as, or at least similar to, your own. Groups provide a forum for the exchange of feelings and ideas, as well as suggestions on how to cope better. Methods of coping and techniques for helping yourself feel better are shared, suggestions are offered, and social relationships can develop. You'll see that you're not alone. This is probably the most important reason for belonging to a group.

These groups are also wonderful for your family, giving family members the chance to get some support of their own. Since one of the best ways to be in control of your emotions is to have a supportive family behind you, you should encourage their participation, too. Do you ever feel shunned or ignored by others (or do you fear feeling this way)? Are your social relationships dwindling? Groups can give you a feeling of belonging.

In groups, any topics you'd like to talk about can be discussed. You may begin to share feelings more openly when you hear others talking about subjects you were previously reluctant to bring up yourself. As a result, a feeling of closeness (almost like family) develops.

Many times, members of groups dealing with chronic medical conditions discuss feelings of hostility toward the medical profession. A person alone with these feelings may have a hard time dealing with physicians and trusting them. In a group, hopefully, the feelings experienced can be straightened out so that a more positive, constructive relationship with a medical professional can be formed.

By the way, there's no law that says that emotional reactions *have* to be shared with others. It's not necessary to talk them out, even though this can be helpful. But these emotional reactions do need to be recognized and worked through. That's the only way to make progress.

Medical Management

Make sure you're getting the best possible medical care. If you haven't already done so, you'll want to establish a good working relationship with a physician. This involves seeing a doctor who not only has expertise in treating MVP but is also understanding, available, and sympathetic to your emotional needs. You'll want to be sure that your physician monitors your condition, so any problems that may arise can be successfully treated. If you're on medication, your physician also must monitor this carefully, so that it is used most effectively and any side effects are minimized.

Medication

You'll frequently hear about medications that improve depression, anxiety, anger, and other emotional problems. Antianxiety medication can be helpful. So can mood elevators and antidepressants. But just remember that your doctor is the one who is in charge of medication. Don't "play with fire."

Psychological Strategies

Professional intervention may be necessary if your emotional problems are severe, or if you want to prevent them from getting worse. Having somebody to talk to can be a big help, especially with a condition like mitral valve prolapse where the symptoms can come and go. Of course, there are some things you can do yourself about your emotions.

HELPING YOURSELF

Let's discuss some of the best techniques you can use to improve the way you feel.

Laugh a Little

Humor can be an amusingly effective way to deal with emotions. Whether it is hearing a joke from someone else, laughing at yourself, or creating your own jokes, humor can be a very relaxing way of dealing with a troublesome situation.

Humor works in three ways. First of all, it reduces anxiety. Laughing is a great way to release tension. Second, it can distract you from those things or feelings that are bothering you. When you're involved in something humorous, you often feel a lot better. Think back, for example, to a time when you were depressed or uncomfortable and somebody asked if you had heard a certain joke. Initially you may have been reluctant to hear it. But before long you were probably totally absorbed in the joke, wondering what the punch line would be! The fact that humor can distract you also means that it can help you to see things from a different perspective. So you may be able to look at something more objectively, which can help you to handle it more effectively.

Finally, the ability to laugh at yourself is a helpful coping strategy. It's also an important part of maturing. How well this works, however, depends on what you're going through. It's just about impossible (and probably ridiculous) to laugh at yourself while you're going through a crisis. However, as you adjust to your condition, you can better use humor as a coping strategy.

Like Yourself

It is often very important for individuals with chronic medical conditions to be "just a little bit more selfish." This is not said in a negative way. But rather, you know yourself and what you need, and it becomes that much more important that you participate in the necessary activities or changes in order to accomplish your needs. This should not be done in a way that is damaging to others. Instead, it should be in a way that states repeatedly to yourself, "I am a worthwhile person and I deserve having nice things in my life." For some people it may be very difficult to learn how to be nice to themselves. For others, they may do so much of it that they may have to temper their enthusiasm so as not to appear to be totally egocentric and self-centered!

What are some of the ways you can be nice to yourself? There are a number of different ways such as buying yourself little goodies, giving yourself some special time to relax, spending time in activities or with people you enjoy, and so on. Everybody has the potential to do plenty of things that they enjoy.

You may want to spend time making a list of those things that would be most interesting and helpful to you. You want to communicate to yourself the message that you are worth it, you are a nice, worthwhile individual, and you deserve nice things. Keep in mind that individuals who are diagnosed with chronic medical problems such as MVP may feel that they have lost some control. Emotionally, they may feel that they are being punished or that bad things are happening to them. It can be very helpful to offset these feeling by reemphasizing the fact that nice things can happen to you.

Being Nice to Others

Sometimes one of the best ways to help your self-esteem is to try to be nice to other people. The feeling of pleasure one gets from helping others can be very gratifying and can help to improve the way you feel about yourself. What are some of the things you can do to be nice to others? You can help virtually any person in virtually any aspect of his or her life, whether it is in home, at work, or recreationally. Visiting people in hospitals, nursing homes, and the like, can be a very easy way to spread sunshine to others. Performing voluntary services in organizations such as churches and schools also can help you to feel good about yourself.

Not only will you feel better about yourself because you'll be helping others, but this will also remind you that you're doing tangible things to better cope with your condition. You'll be feeling more productive. You'll feel more like you belong and are a part of society. You'll find a number of different outlets in your life that will help you to reduce boredom.

Relaxation Procedures

Relaxation is the opposite of tension. So if you learn to relax, you'll be much less tense. But relaxation procedures, by themselves, will not totally control your emotions. So why use them? Because if you're feeling more relaxed, you'll be better able to identify those problems that are affecting you, and you'll then be better able to figure out how to deal with them. Relaxation procedures, then, can be an essential first step in coping with your emotions.

How do you relax? We're talking about clinical relaxation, now— not everyday activities like reading, gardening, listening to music, or sitting in front of the television with a can of beer! There are different types of clinical relaxation procedures. For example, progressive relaxation is a procedure in which you learn how to relax the muscles in your body. Hypnosis is another relaxation procedure, as is meditation and the "relaxation response." There's also a procedure called imagery, in which you view pictures in your mind that will help to relax you, thereby making it easier for you to solve problems. (More information about imagery can be found in the later chapter on Pain.) Books on any of these procedures are available in your local library, and can really help you to start feeling better.

Here's a quick introduction to one relaxation procedure. I call it, appropriately, the "quick release." Read the directions first and then try it. Close your eyes, take a deep breath, and hold it as you tighten every muscle in your body that you can think of (your fists, arms, legs, stomach, neck, buttocks, etc.). Hold your breath, keeping your muscles tense, for about six seconds. Then let it out in a "whoosh," and allow the tension to drain out of your muscles. Let your body go limp. Keep your eyes closed, and breathe rhythmically and comfortably for about twenty seconds. Repeat this tension-relaxation cycle three times. By the end of the third repetition, you'll probably feel a lot more relaxed.

Pinpointing

Are you more comfortable now? Then you're ready to proceed to the next crucial step. In order to deal with anything that's upsetting you, you'll want to determine exactly what it is that's bothering you! Make a list of these things. Then go over what you've written. In reviewing your list you'll see that just about every item can be placed into one of two categories. The first category contains the modifiables, or the things (whether problems or emotions) you *can* do something about. The second category includes the nonmodifiables, or things you can't do anything about. Why separate them? Because the two categories have different implications for strategies you can use to deal with them.

For the first category, you'll want to figure out what techniques you can use to improve the situation. You'll plan a course of action as soon as you identify exactly what's bothering you. How about the second category? You'll still be planning strategies, but of a different kind! Where do your emotions exist? In your mind, right? Therefore, your plan for this category is to work on the way you're thinking.

What Should You Do?

How can you change your thinking so that something will bother you less? The technique you use really depends on what emotional reaction is bothering you. For example, if you're afraid of something and you want to conquer this fear, a procedure called systematic desensitization may be helpful. We'll go into this later in the chapter on Fears and Anxieties.

If you're feeling guilty or angry about something, or if something is depressing you, it can be very helpful for you to learn how to change or "restructure" the way you're thinking. You'll learn more about techniques for that in the later chapters on Guilt, Anger, and Depression.

Actually, any of the procedures we've discussed can be used with just about any problem. It's just a question of deciding what's best for *you* in how you cope with your emotions.

WHAT ABOUT THE FUTURE?

Even if you do have intense emotional reactions, these will diminish, either because of the passage of time or because you're doing something to help. On the other hand, you'll experience more emotional reactions when your symptoms are more pronounced. So you'll probably experience a range of emotional reactions from time to time. But even when these feelings do occur, you can usually point to so many positive things going on in your life—so many ways that you can recognize progress—that it may not be such a difficult thing to deal with. That's how to develop the positive mental attitude that you want to be an integral part of your life.

Although emotions do not cause MVP, they can certainly interfere with your ability to live with it. In addition, emotional upsets can, in some cases, exacerbate your condition. So doesn't it make sense to do what you can to control your emotions?

The purpose of this section is to help you to understand the different emotions you may experience. You'll discover where they come from and, very importantly, recognize that many others have gone through exactly what you're going through. In addition, a number of strategies will be presented to help you cope with these emotions more effectively. Remember that "practice makes better." Just reading about a method to control an emotion doesn't mean you'll experience instant success. You have to keep practicing.

In the following chapters you'll see how these different techniques can be used. So don't be afraid, depressed, angry, or guilty! Instead, read on!

6

Coping With the Diagnosis

Yes, this chapter is called "Coping With the Diagnosis." But, you may say, I had trouble coping before I was even diagnosed! Many people have had strange experiences that other people just do not understand. Did people ever tell you, "It's all in your head," because of the symptoms you've described, or the experiences you've had? Have you ever been a "doctor shopper"? This might be because you know you're feeling something, but it doesn't matter whom you go to, you don't feel you're getting the correct answers.

Have you felt that you're not meeting physicians who really understand or are able to help with what you need help with? Have you been on a number of different types of medications, hoping something, sometime, will help you to deal with your symptoms?

Have you been told that you have psychiatric problems, and that the problems are all in your head? Have you had difficulties with jobs or your marriage because of the fatigue or other anxiety symptoms that you may experience because of the condition? Many people with MVP have reported similar experiences. It may have been very unpleasant for you to go through these things, but isn't it nicer to know that you weren't the only one!

INITIAL REACTIONS

When you first found out you had MVP, how did you feel? How did you react when your doctor finally told you the news? When first diagnosed, some people may not even react, since it still may not be "real" to them. But others go through a hard time. You may know someone who has MVP, or have heard about the experiences of some people with the condition. Perhaps this frightened you. Emotional reactions to mitral valve prolapse are not always rational. As a matter of fact, in many cases they are completely irrational. As the full impact of the diagnosis sets in, you may experience a whole variety of emotional reactions, ranging from sadness and anxiety to anger, frustration, and despair.

Not only can the diagnosis of MVP, and the time afterward, be frightening, but many people who have been diagnosed have become withdrawn. Why? They may be more reluctant to share what they are experiencing with people for fear of getting responses indicating disbelief. It became more important to get information about MVP, or at least some kind of validation that could be shared with family and friends who have grown not to believe them. And, of course, they wanted to get some answers that would help them to solve the problem.

Many people who are diagnosed with MVP experience two completely different types of reactions.

Reaction 1: What a Relief!

One type of reaction is that of relief. Now, that may seem strange to you! Why would you be relieved to know that you have MVP? Well, perhaps you were experiencing a lot of chest pain and nothing seemed to help. Maybe you were frightened that you were "having the big one!" Certain symptoms may have really frightened you. You might have thought you had major heart problems, or some other fatal problem (some people actually feel this way!). Wow, were you relieved to find out that you weren't dying!

Maybe you've gone from doctor to doctor, trying to find out what was really wrong with you, so you could begin a treatment plan that would finally help you to feel better. Maybe physicians or your family and friends didn't believe you, and thought the problem was all in your head! That can really be annoying! If things had gone on indefinitely, you might have started wondering yourself (or maybe you already *did* wonder)!

At last, the correct diagnosis was made. Knowing the cause can be a relief. If you were relieved after your diagnosis, you probably had a much easier time coping early on. Why? One reason is because you're hopeful that treatment will improve the way you've been feeling (and it's good to finally know why you're feeling that way). Second, family members and friends who may not have believed that you were really sick will now discover that there has been some truth to your physical complaints. Unfortunately, some people close to you still may not believe that the problem is physical. They may continue to believe that the problem is either emotional or stress-related. You can't force everyone to believe a medical diagnosis! However, most doubts probably will disappear. Strained relationships may improve. Family members may sometimes feel guilty as they realize that they have been skeptical about your condition. They may have criticized your inability to fulfill responsibilities and your decreased ability to do things. They did this because they thought a real problem did not exist. Now they know the truth! Third, and most important, you'll be relieved that it wasn't all in your head. After a long period of time, even the most confident person can begin to wonder whether or not there is really something wrong or if it is purely emotional.

Reaction 2: Panic Attack!

The other reaction (certainly not a pleasant one) is terror. Sheer panic! You might have reacted, "Oh, no, I have a problem with my heart! What is it? Where does it come from? Why do I have it? I'm too young for this!" Or you may ask, "What's going to happen to me?"; "How will MVP affect me?"; "Will I ever be 'normal?'"; "What is the treatment (and how will I handle it)?"; "Am I going to have a heart attack?"; "Will I ever get better?"; "Who will take care of me?"; "Am I going to die?" These are all tense questions that may pop up when you're diagnosed. Family members and loved ones may ask them (and panic) as well. You may think that your life may never be the same again. For life will now include MVP.

Let's talk about this reaction. Does anyone you know like having a chronic medical problem or physical restrictions? No way. It's normal to be upset and afraid. You probably don't understand the diagnosis (and how many of you knew about MVP beforehand?).

After all, mitral valve prolapse even sounds frightening!

You may suddenly be hit with the fact that you are mortal and vulnerable. You'll realize you may have this problem for the rest of your life. Physically, it's not uncommon to feel faint, dizzy, or to experience other stress reactions at the time of diagnosis.

WHY MIGHT I FEEL CALM?

Frequently, as with any traumatic event, you may feel numb at first. You may sit quietly in the doctor's office, listening to everything that is being said. But you may not really be absorbing it. You may hear your doctor talking, even hear the reassuring words, but his words are not penetrating. You might even actively and calmly participate in the discussion, without any emotional reaction. That may come later!

HOW ABOUT DENIAL?

Denying that a problem exists is not unusual. Regardless of what symptoms you've been experiencing, hearing that you have mitral valve prolapse may provoke denial. You may protest, "Oh, you're just making that up," "I don't have this problem the way you think I do," "Why don't you give it a little more time; I'm sure the problem will go away by itself," or even "#!(*) x#, leave me alone!"

If you're reading this book, then chances are you're probably not denying your condition. But if you are denying, the best way to start coping with your situation is to face reality. Speak to those professionals who know about MVP and have them explain it in further detail. Let them explain why treatment is necessary. Read about, or talk to, other people with MVP and listen to what they went through when they were first diagnosed. You will find that many of their experiences parallel your own.

Did you ever ask yourself, "Why can't I go back to the way things used to be?" Have you ever wished you could wake up one morning and find out that this was all a bad dream? The more you keep hoping that it will go away, the more you are slowing down your adjustment. Why is this so? Because you're not really admitting to yourself that you've changed, perhaps permanently. Rather, you're trying to push it out of your mind, hoping that things will return to the way they were. Such denial can obviously make it hard to cope with having MVP, since the problem is not being faced realistically. Try to recognize that your condition does exist now, that it affects you, and that it will remain with you. Try to plan all your activities and aim all your thinking toward the notion that you are going to do what you can to handle it effectively.

HOW DO YOU START TO ADJUST?

You must help yourself. Sure, you can receive love and support from your family and friends, and you can get expertise and support from professionals. But that's never enough. You are the one who is going to have to come to grips with MVP. This is something you have to do yourself, regardless of what anyone else says or does. At first, adjusting may be a difficult struggle. It may require a lot of effort and understanding. You may go through a lot of emotional turmoil, but there is no other way out. You must face it.

Information, please! Get as much of it as you can. Most of your initial reactions probably occurred because you didn't know enough about MVP. So you'll want to learn as much as possible. Your physician will be helpful in suggesting ways of getting current information.

After reading general, consumer-oriented information, you might want to move on to more technical material. Ask questions about anything you don't understand. And certainly ask questions about anything that frightens you. After all, medical writing is not designed to calm down the person with MVP. It will just state medical facts and statistics. If you forget this, it would be easy to get frightened!

It probably wasn't a lifelong goal of yours to become an expert on MVP, but think about how much this can help you. Doctors will respect your questions more. And you'll understand exactly what's going on in your body. These are just two of the many advantages that can come from reading about your condition.

DEALING WITH YOUR EMOTIONAL REACTIONS

Begin working consciously to control any anxiety or stress that's making you feel less than comfortable. Once you have accepted the fact that you have MVP, you'll start determining in which ways (if any) you'll have to alter your lifestyle. In addition, you'll want to try to control as many harmful emotions as you can.

It's very easy for your imagination to run wild. Initially, you'll probably keep thinking about all the things that can possibly go wrong. You'll worry about every symptom. You also may get frightened about how serious MVP could get, and how it can affect you and the people close to you. So learn the facts about your condition. This is a great way to alleviate some of the anxiety caused by the diagnosis. Learn as much as you can.

The emotions stemming from the diagnosis of MVP can be unpleasant. You may experience regret, sorrow, and nostalgia, remembering the way it used to be. Many fears may come to mind, some of which can be overwhelming. Fear of incapacitation, of having a heart attack, of losing friends, are all very common fears. Begin facing them. They can and must be faced in order to move your adjustment along more smoothly. Speak to other people who have MVP. Learn how they've adjusted. This can be very helpful.

WHAT'S NEXT?

Once you've become more familiar with your condition and understand how it affects you, what can you do to deal with it? For one thing, learn what specific changes may have to be made in your lifestyle. There is no way of knowing how many changes you'll have to make, but you do want to create the best possible life for yourself.

Obviously, work with a physician you can trust, one who has had experience working with people with MVP before. Many people with MVP work with a cardiologist. But others, especially if symptoms are mild, may work with their internists, family doctors, or whomever. Of course, you may work with doctors in other specialties as well, depending on your symptoms. But they all should be doctors you're comfortable with and have confidence in.

You have the right to learn as much as possible about the different treatments for MVP. How do you find out? Start by asking questions of your physician. Remember, the patient-physician relationship is very important in MVP, as it is in any chronic medical problem. If your physician does not seem receptive to your questions, then you may have to reconsider this relationship.

Because your medical problem is ongoing, your relationship with your physician will be ongoing as well. There will be much more contact than you would normally have with your physician if you didn't have MVP. Some say this relationship is like a marriage (but unfortunately, you're not entitled to 50 percent of your doctor's assets if you separate!).

HOW ABOUT THE FAMILY?

A very important part of adjusting to the diagnosis of MVP is for your family to learn to adjust as well. It's hard for everyone if those around you have difficulty accepting your condition. But dealing with the diagnosis can be hard for family members. They, too, will go through periods of denial when they will say, "No, everything will be fine, " or "I'm sure the problem will clear up by itself."

Jeanette, a twenty-nine-year-old teacher, had only recently been diagnosed as having mitral valve prolapse. After a few depressing weeks, however, she began to learn how to cope. She was finally able to handle thoughts of lifestyle changes, concerns about reduced energy, and some of the other unpleasant thoughts associated with MVP. Sound great? Not really. You see, her husband of eight years couldn't accept the fact that she had a problem, her children were afraid she was going to die, and her fifty-eight-year-old mother had contacted virtually every cardiologist from New York to Alaska! Although Jeanette was learning how to cope with MVP, she could not cope with her family. They couldn't handle it, and were making things very difficult for her.

It's a great idea for family members to seek out people to speak to. They, too, can find out more about MVP and about how others cope with treatment. Family members can follow the same suggestions given before: seeking information, speaking to physicians, and talking to others. So encourage family members and any willing friends to learn as much as they can. This will help your adjustment.

IN A NUTSHELL

Start thinking positively about your life with MVP. Learn as much as you can about your condition. Use whatever support systems are necessary to help you. Use all the stress management and emotional control procedures available. Start saying to yourself, "MVP may be part of me, but I'm still alive and I'm going to do whatever I can to help myself adjust to this." If it's necessary for you to make changes in your lifestyle, even major ones, tell yourself that you will make them, and you will make them willingly! You are going to lead as complete a life as you can. The more quickly you can adjust your lifestyle to fit your needs, the more rapidly you will be able to enjoy your life. This may be hard at first and will take time. But at least be grateful that you're not helpless and can take steps to make the most of your life with MVP!

7

Depression

Marian felt very blue. A thirty-five-year-old mother of three, married for twelve years, living in a comfortable home in a good neighborhood, she apparently had everything she could ask for, except for mitral valve prolapse. She didn't ask for that. She found herself feeling increasingly upset with the changes that had to be made in her life. She felt that she got tired too easily; she felt afraid that her life would be shorter. She didn't have enough energy for her children. She felt helpless and hopeless. Marian was suffering from depression.

Depression is a serious problem. The very mention of the word can sometimes knock the smile right off your face. Actual numbers vary, but it is estimated that more than two million Americans need professional care for depression. Because it is so widespread, depression has been nicknamed the "common cold" of emotional problems.

Just what is depression? Depression is an extremely unpleasant feeling of unhappiness and despair. It can range from mild (where you may feel discouraged and downhearted) to severe (where you can feel utterly hopeless, worthless, and unwilling to go on living). You may feel that there is no reason to remain a part of the world.

Depression can be painful. Imagine how it must hurt to feel (or say), "I wish I were never born. What good am I? I'm not helping anybody around me and I'm not helping myself." It may seem like life and the world are against you. Life is unfair. It is a constant struggle in which you never win. That hurts.

DEPRESSION AFFECTS YOUR BODY

The more noticeable symptoms of depression may be physical. Nervous activity or agitation, such as wringing of the hands, may occur. You may be restless, or have difficulty remaining in one place. Or, on the other hand, you may become much less active, and remain motionless for abnormally long periods of time (appearing almost in a trance, with no apparent desire to do anything). Jim became very concerned when his twenty-eight-year-old wife, Jane, remained sitting in a chair in the living room for hours at a time. When he asked her a question she would respond in monosyllables. When friends called on the phone, she never wanted to talk to them. Jane's depression was causing her to lose interest in just about everything.

Other physical changes that can occur if you're depressed are a reduction or increase in appetite, a decreased interest in sex, and, for some women, cessation of menstruation. If you're mildly depressed, you may have difficulty concentrating, and your attention span may be much shorter. Men may remain unshaven simply because they don't feel like shaving. When you speak (and you'll probably do less of that, too) your conversation will usually be shallow, emphasizing feelings of worthlessness and despair. Most of your physical activities will also slow down (and not just because of mitral valve prolapse restrictions).

You'll probably feel exhausted. This may seem surprising, since you're not doing much of anything anyway. But constantly telling yourself that you're no good can be very tiring! You really don't want to believe this, but you feel like you have no choice. In attempting to escape these feelings you may become even more depressed, as well as more physically drained and exhausted.

Depression may cause you to feel physically sick. This is because of the many ways your body reacts when you're depressed. Any of the depressive symptoms we've talked about thus far might be related to a physical disorder. But if the symptoms go away when your depression improves, don't just assume that they're related to the depression. A medical examination may still be a good idea. This way, you'll be sure that there is no organic disease causing your depression.

DEPRESSION AFFECTS YOUR MOOD

You may experience frequent mood swings. For example, you might feel worse in the morning and better in the evening. This may be because of a number of reasons. For example, you may realize that it's almost time to go to sleep—a means of escape. But depression also may cause difficulty sleeping, even if you weren't doing much of anything during the day.

When you're depressed, you feel like your mood keeps getting "lower." You like yourself very little, if at all. Your thinking is very negative, very different from the way it is when you're feeling good.

It is your negative thinking (not just a particular triggering event) that leads to your depression. This negative thinking tends to be the most frequently overlooked and misunderstood part of depression. Recognizing this is an important first step in learning to cope with depression.

DEPRESSION AFFECTS RELATIONSHIPS WITH OTHERS

If you're depressed, you may feel that people around you have no need for you. You may feel that others consider you to be an uninteresting, boring person.

Do you feel less at ease talking to others? Does it seem like others are having a hard time talking to you, even if they have been close to you for a long time? Because of your depression, you may be less interested in conversation and less confident. You may project your feelings of self-worthlessness onto others, believing that they really don't want to talk to you. The more depressed you are, the more persuasive you may be in convincing other people around you that you're no good.

Bernadette received a telephone call from her friend Tina. Tina wanted to know how Bernadette had been feeling, since the last time they had gotten together Bernadette seemed to be very tired, and experiencing a lot of chest pain. Bernadette responded half-heartedly, imagining that Tina was only calling out of obligation. She then explained that she would understand if Tina did not want to call again, since she never seemed to have any good news to tell her. How do you think Tina felt? Imagine hearing this repeatedly, despite reassuring Bernadette that her concern was sincere. Would you be surprised if, eventually, Tina got tired of even trying, and probably stopped calling? But in Bernadette's mind, this would only reinforce the fact that she really was no good, and that she was not worthy of having any friends after all!

DEPRESSION AFFECTS PHYSICAL ACTIVITIES

Do you find that you are getting less satisfaction from the normal activities you can participate in? Are you functioning like a robot? Does it seem like something is missing? It can be depressing to realize that something you used to enjoy no longer gives you the same pleasure, especially if you don't know why. It may almost seem like there is a force propelling you to "go through the motions," while your heart just isn't in it. It is understandable, therefore, that if you are depressed, you might prefer to withdraw from such activities.

WHAT KICKS OFF DEPRESSION?

A bout of depression frequently seems to start with one specific thing, an event or occurrence that makes you unhappy. Gloria had been planning a big dinner party for over two months. Although she had been more tired recently, she still was able to go with a friend to buy a beautiful cocktail dress. In the weeks prior to the party, she tried to get as much rest as possible. The big day finally came. Gloria felt so physically weak that she had to talk herself into getting through it. She tried to think about seeing friends and relatives, the money she had spent on her dress, and the feeling that she did not want to give in to her MVP. But what happened? She had no choice but to sit the entire evening because she was just too weak to get up. When the party was over, she was so depressed and weak that she remained in bed, crying and miserable, for over a week. That one evening triggered a long depression. She felt like even the most important things to her were ruined because of mitral valve prolapse.

What happens after that first depressing event occurs? A kind of chain reaction follows. This one occurrence creates a feeling that spreads like wildfire. It's almost as if the bottom has dropped out of your world. You may feel less able to control your thinking (although this is not true, as we will see later). But keep in mind: the deeper you go into depression, the harder it is to climb back out again. Therefore, you certainly want to catch these feelings of depression as early as possible, to try to keep yourself from spiraling further downward.

WHAT CAUSES DEPRESSION?

Where does depression come from? Sometimes we can figure this out, and sometimes we can't. But before we give up, let's discuss some of the possible causes.

How About the Normal "Downs"?

A certain amount of depression is normal in anyone's life. Nobody's life is a constant "upper." We all experience normal cycles of ups and downs. If we never experienced some of the downs, how could we ever fully appreciate the ups?! However, when depression becomes more than just the "normal downs," then it must be attended to. Nipping it quickly in the bud can keep it from becoming much worse.

There are certain things in anyone's life that can understandably lead to depression. Certain traumatic experiences such as losing a loved one, being diagnosed with a chronic medical problem, requiring major surgery, being fired from a job, all may certainly lead to depression. That's understandable. However, this doesn't mean you should ignore the problem or wait until it goes away. It's essential to learn how to deal with depression, since this is so important in learning how to cope with mitral valve prolapse.

How About Anger You Can't Express?

What if you get so angry that you feel like you're going to burst? But you don't (or can't) do anything about it, so you decide to "swallow" it. It seems strange that a powerful feeling like anger can turn into a withdrawn, helpless feeling like depression. But it's true. If you become increasingly angry about something and feel unable to do anything about it, you may turn the anger inward. You may feel so much frustration or hopelessness that you "shut down" in an attempt to keep yourself from these terrible feelings. This leads to withdrawal, which is a symptom of depression.

Is It All in Our Minds?

A small percentage of depression cases may be caused by biochemical deficiencies—some chemical imbalance in our bodies. This does not occur very often, however. Treatment for biochemical deficiencies may involve the administration of drugs in an effort to rebalance the chemicals in our bodies. This usually isn't the whole answer. But regardless of whether your depression is caused by this or, more typically, by your reactions to things, people, and events around you, you should still try to modify your behavior and improve your thinking. Many experts believe that even if the cause of depression is biochemical, by working on improving your thoughts and behaviors you can have a positive effect on your depression.

How About Mitral Valve Prolapse?

Can MVP cause depression? Are you kidding??? Knowing you have a problem with your mitral valve can certainly create depression or magnify already-existing depression.

The depression you felt after being diagnosed with MVP is understandable. But it can (and should) get better as you begin to adjust to your new life situation. There's a problem, though. Because life with mitral valve prolapse has its ups and downs (physically), your feelings may bounce up and down as well. This can be a problem, considering what depression can do to you. So, it's worth learning how to cope with depression.

You may be saying to yourself, "If I'm depressed over my MVP, how can I expect to get over my depression unless my MVP is cured?" That kind of thinking will get you nowhere. You know that your mitral valve prolapse is a chronic condition. So if your depression lingers, don't wait. Work on it. Learn how to cope with it. We'll talk more later about how you can improve your thinking.

What else about mitral valve prolapse might depress you? You might become depressed thinking about the future, not knowing how MVP will affect your life. Changes in habits necessitated by your condition and its treatment may also be depressing. You might get depressed because of (or as a result of) having to take medications.

Problems involving other people may depress you. You may feel helpless at not being able to share what you're experiencing or the way you feel. You may get depressed if others don't understand what you're going through (not that you want to be pitied, though!). People may expect more from you than you're able to (or want to) provide. You may be depressed over the possibility of damaged relationships, lost friendships, or family friction. If you're single, you may become depressed thinking that you'll never meet anyone (not that there need be any truth to this at all!).

Depression can result from changes in lifestyle. You might not be able to participate in activities you used to love. You might have to change your work routine, as well as your family routine. Money problems, with no immediate solution imminent, can certainly be depressing. Just having mitral valve prolapse, with its intangible effects on your day-to-day living, can get to you.

WHAT MAINTAINS DEPRESSION?

You may be blaming yourself (or your MVP) for everything that is wrong. You may tend to become more and more withdrawn, and pull away from the world around you. Why? Well, if you believe that your condition is causing all these horrible things, isn't it better to "escape" and not think about it? Realistically, escaping doesn't solve anything. But if you're depressed, you may feel that withdrawal is the only way to solve this dilemma. This keeps you depressed (in fact, it can make you even more depressed).

Although you may seem sullen and withdrawn to others, you're probably in deep emotional pain. Part of what makes you, and keeps you, depressed is your failure to protect yourself from this emotional pain. When your mind does allow any thoughts to enter, you tend to feel overwhelmed by feelings of doom and destruction. You feel that nothing good can possibly happen, that only bad things can happen. So what do you do? You try to block everything out of your mind!

So why do you stay depressed? Why doesn't it just go away? It may be because you don't want to talk to anybody, or to even consider therapy. Therefore, the thoughts and feelings leading to your depression tend to be kept hidden. You may ask, "Is my unwillingness to talk the only reason why I'm still depressed? If I start talking more, will that get me out of my depression?" Not necessarily. But it can be helpful to talk out your feelings. It probably would be helpful (even though you wouldn't be too thrilled) if a close friend or family member took the initiative and forced you into some kind of conversation (therapeutic or otherwise) or, at least, into doing something constructive.

HOW DO WE DEAL WITH DEPRESSION?

Can anything be done? Of course! Would I abandon you without any suggestions? First, tell yourself that the main reason why you're still depressed is because you have not yet taken the proper steps toward feeling better! These steps can "bring you out of the rut" and reacquaint you with the more positive, pleasant aspects of living that you'd like to experience. Don't think it's easy, though. Unfortunately, once you've fallen into depression, it takes effort, hard work, and a certain amount of persistence to pull yourself back up. The fight, however, is surely worth it. Of course, the fight can be made easier if you know of specific techniques and activities that will help.

Once you feel better, you're not ever going to want to feel that depressed again, right? Well, the strategies and techniques that are most effective in dealing with depression also can be effective in preventing you from becoming depressed again! This doesn't mean you'll never feel depressed again. It may happen. Anticipate it, so that if it does recur, you won't completely fall apart. And if it does happen, won't it be good to know that you can fight it? You *can* do something to help yourself!

Depression Treatment

Now that you're ready to fight your depression, consider two major ways of dealing with it: being more physical (in other words, doing something), and working on your thinking.

It can be very helpful to make a list of all the things that are depressing you. You may feel there'll be at least fifty items! But in actuality, you'll probably start running out of ideas after six or seven. Then divide this list into two more lists: first, things that you can do something about, and second, things you can't do anything about. (Sound familiar?) You read about this earlier. But it really works for a number of different problems. Get physical (do something) about those items in the first list, and get thoughtful (work on your thinking) regarding those items in the second list.

Let's Get Physical

Unknowingly, you may be using a lot of energy to keep yourself depressed. You may be working hard to keep that anger inside, even if it appears to others that you are withdrawing. If your depression is anger turned within, then we can logically assume that, by releasing it, feelings of depression can be eliminated. But what do you do with those feelings? You must find an object toward which your anger can be expressed. This may be difficult. However, it's important to release the trapped anger so that it doesn't build up further and deepen the depression.

Have you ever been in this situation? You're sitting there, depressed and withdrawn. Somebody makes an innocent remark, and you practically snap the person's head off! What's happening? Whatever was said triggered the release of the internalized anger that was making you depressed. Look out, world!

Consider for a moment all the energy that is keeping you depressed. You've read about why it is important to release this energy outwardly. What kinds of activities can be helpful for this? Many types of intense physical activity can release this energy. But although getting physical may improve your depression, it's your thoughts that make you depressed. Physical activity can provide a great distraction, which can help you to look more objectively at what's going on. That will help. But it may not teach you what you need the most: ways of fighting inappropriate thinking. Besides, mitral valve prolapse may not even allow you to participate in intense physical activity! Fortunately, this isn't the only way to lift depression.

Let's Get Thoughtful

If you can "think" yourself into depression, you can obviously "think" yourself out of it. How? Your thoughts show how you "talk to yourself." In fact, when it comes to talking to yourself, you're probably the biggest chatterbox you know! But if you're depressed, you're just talking yourself down. All your comments (or at least most of them) are probably put-downs: harsh statements offering little to be happy about. These can make you feel even worse. You want your inner voice to help you, not hurt you. Let's see how you can do that.

Distinguishing Fact From Fiction

Don't get defensive when I tell you this: When you're depressed, you tend to distort reality. Clinical research with depressed patients has proven this. Recognize, therefore, that your thoughts are not necessarily based on what is really going on, but on your own distorted views. This is called cognitive distortion.

Is that bad? You bet your happiness it is. "Cognitive" refers to your thinking. "Distortion" means you're twisting things around and, in general, losing sight of what's real. We all tend to do this from time to time. But when you're depressed, you do it a lot, if not all the time, and it keeps you depressed. So how do you stop? First, you must become reacquainted with what is really happening and with the facts. But how can you do that if you keep distorting reality? Right now, you're better off accepting somebody else's perceptions of the situation, because that person is probably a lot more objective and accurate. Since so many feelings of worthlessness are based on distorted facts, depression can be reduced, if not eliminated, once these facts are straightened out.

Angela kept moaning because none of her friends were calling her. "They don't call as much as they used to. I guess they just don't care." Her sister, Stephanie, asked her to estimate how often her friends used to call. When Angela compared this number to the current number of calls she was receiving, she realized that the numbers were almost the same. She then realized that she was probably just more sensitive because of all the changes going on in her life! Although she did not feel 100 percent better, it was good to know that she wasn't being abandoned.

Making Molehills Out of Mountains

Does this imply that if you're depressed you have no real problems? Is it "all in your head"? No. Everyone has problems. If you feel good, you can handle them, but if you're depressed, you may feel overwhelmed. Each and every part of your life, regardless of how trivial or slight it may be, tends to depress you. As the depression lifts, you will again be able to deal with all of life's problems, big and small.

Self-Fulfilling Prophecy

We've discussed several different ways that you may feel if you're depressed. Are all these feelings irrational and untrue? No. Ironically, although some of them may start off being far from the truth, the longer you feel that way the more chance there will be for them to become "self-fulfilling prophecies." In other words, you'll begin convincing yourself that nonsense makes sense. For example, if you begin telling yourself that friends and relatives don't care, this may become a reality because your negative attitudes may alienate the people close to you. They may decide it's not worth the bother. As far as your activities go, you are less likely to do anything when you're depressed. You'll probably be less likely to even attempt doing things that you used to enjoy. As a result, you'll feel less competent and will not accomplish anything. This just tends to magnify and confirm your feelings of worthlessness, leading to even greater depression. Not a pretty picture.

Once you begin feeling depressed, your negative thoughts will soon lead to negative actions. These negative actions will lead to more negative thoughts, which will in turn lead to more negative actions, and so on. It is an ongoing, vicious circle that will spiral you further downward into deeper depression. Eventually you'll feel trapped in this vicious circle, with no way to escape from the "dumps."

Are you getting depressed just reading this? In all probability, if you've ever been depressed, you've said to yourself at least once already, "Wow, that sounds just like me!" So you see, your negative thoughts become self-fulfilling prophecies. If you find that you are starting to believe in your negative thoughts, stop yourself. Try to think positive thoughts, so that if your thought does turn out to be real, it will at least be a positive one.

Positive is the Opposite of Negative

As we've said before, depression results from and causes a lot of negative thinking. Negative thoughts automatically pop into your mind and you cannot stop them. It's like trying to keep your eyes open when you sneeze! You just can't do it. But once you become aware of them, then you can do something. People who remain depressed feel incapable of doing anything about their negative thinking and allow these thoughts to continue. They simply continue in that vicious, downward circle that was mentioned earlier.

Ann, a thirty-four-year-old housewife, was resting when the telephone rang. "I'm sure that's Katherine, calling to cancel our lunch plans," she sadly thought to herself. Within the thirty seconds it took her to get to the phone, she had become so depressed that she considered not even answering the call. Imagine how she felt when she reluctantly answered the phone and discovered that it was a wrong number! Ann had allowed her negative thoughts to run wild—

she became more and more negative until she was about ready to give up. And for what? There was no clear-cut reason for thinking the way she did.

Once she realized that she was thinking this way, what should she have done? She should have countered her thoughts. She should have told herself, "It may not even be Katherine on the phone. Or if it is, maybe she's just calling to confirm. I won't let it bother me now. After all, I don't even know who it is!" This is the beginning of positive thinking.

Dwell on the Brighter Tomorrows

Wanda was depressed because she constantly compared her present condition to the way she used to be. She was afraid to swim (an activity that she loved), stay out late with her girlfriends, spend hours in museums, or participate in other favorite strenuous activities. She allowed these depressing thoughts to overwhelm her, and as a result, certainly did not give herself a chance to enjoy her life.

If you find yourself unhappily comparing your present life to life before MVP, try to modify your thinking. Start planning fun things for the present and future. Anyone can come up with some enjoyable things to do, regardless of any physical restrictions. But it takes effort. Don't wallow in self-pity, because that will allow your depression to strangle you. Work on your thinking, develop some positive plans, and translate them into pleasure. Then wave good-bye to your depression!

When you recall the past, you may not even think it was that much better. You may have had other physical problems. You may have made some mistakes in your life. This may make you even more depressed about the future. However, you can't change the past. What's done is done. Keep telling yourself that. Tell yourself that you're going to work on making the future better. Set up some specific goals, starting with the easy-to-reach ones. You'll be helping yourself just by thinking about what you can do that's more positive. Don't punish yourself for the past.

What's Missing From Your Life?

You may have laughed when you read the title of this section. "Good health," you might respond. "A properly closing mitral valve!" Sure.

But why discuss this? Because depressed people frequently lament the fact that something is missing from their lives. What is usually missing is a feeling of satisfaction, accomplishment, and pride that normally comes from others' praise. You may just miss the attention and interest of other people. This may cause you to feel worthless. How do you counteract this? Think about your positive qualities (yes, you do have some!). Think about how you can interact more with people, spark their interest, and obtain more of the satisfaction that makes you feel worthwhile.

Shoot for the Earth, Not the Moon

We all have goals for ourselves. It's normal to become depressed when we don't reach a particular goal, especially if we've tried very hard to get there. But maybe it's not a realistic goal. Maybe you're trying to do something you can't, and you're getting depressed instead of realistically resetting your goal.

If your goals are more realistically set, you'll have a much better chance of achieving them, and less of a chance of falling short.

AN ANTI-DEPRESSING SUMMARY

The best way to work on negative thoughts is to prevent them from continuing. Be more realistically positive. Deal with reality the way it actually exists. Deal with thoughts from a more factual point of view. Deal with them the way somebody else might—somebody who is not depressed and who can be more objective. Try to make your perceptions more accurate, your awareness more realistic, and your thoughts more positive and constructive. Remember: Your thoughts lead to your emotions. If your thoughts are negative and critical, then your emotions also will be in bad shape. If you can turn your thoughts around to a more positive, constructive point of view, you'll see that your emotional reactions will improve as well.

8

Fears and Anxieties

Don't be "afraid" to read this chapter! It may help you discover what you're "anxious" about!

The two sentences above may help you to distinguish between fear and anxiety. What's the difference? Anxiety is a general sense of uneasiness: a vague feeling of discomfort. It is an agitated, uncertain state in which you just don't feel at peace or in control. There is a premonition that something bad may happen, which you have to protect yourself against. You feel very vulnerable. However, you're not exactly sure what the source of your anxiety is.

Fear, on the other hand, is usually more specific. It's often directed toward something that can be recognized, whether it's a person, object, situation, or event. We have fear when we become aware of something dangerous, or when we feel threatened. When we are afraid (as with feeling anxious) we also feel out of control and less confident. So the feelings of fear and anxiety are basically the same. The main difference is whether you can identify the source of the feeling. From this point on, however, I'll be using the two terms interchangeably so there is less confusion.

Fear is so prevalent that many words are used to describe it: scared, concerned, alarmed, worried, uptight, nervous, edgy, and shaky. Then there's perplexed, wary, frightened, helpless, and frustrated. Is that it? Nope! How about suspicious, keyed-up, impatient, giddy, hesitant, apprehensive, tense, panicky, disturbed, and agitated? Of course, there are more, but if I went on, this book would have to be renamed "The Fear Synonym Book." All these words mean the same thing: "I'm afraid." The source of this fear may be real or imaginary.

FEAR AND MVP

Unfortunately, fear and anxiety can be a "too common" experience for individuals who have MVP. This may be for either of two reasons. First, it may be because of the concerns you have because you have the condition. Or second, maybe you were one of many people who have been misdiagnosed as having an anxiety disorder or a panic disorder, instead of the correct diagnosis of MVP Syndrome. Frustrating, right?

Because anxiety is often such a common, unpleasant part of MVP, and because anxiety can interfere with your ability to best deal with any medical problem, this really is something important to work on.

Anxiety is a very complex phenomenon. It can include psychological, biological, and social components. It certainly is not surprising that if you have symptoms such as shortness of breath, chest pain, or palpitations, you'll be frightened by these symptoms! This anxiety may lead to biochemical responses that may only cause things to get worse.

Despite years of experience of living with MVP, there are many people who will still become frightened when they first feel a chest pain. This fear can be much more pronounced when it occurs at night or, as it does for many people, when it awakens them from a deep sleep. Nighttime can be a more frightening time in general. When you experience chest pain at night, the fear may be more pronounced. Why? You might be worrying about a heart attack, as well as the lack of availability of supportive family or professionals during the wee hours.

WHAT DOES ANXIETY FEEL LIKE?

What happens when you get extremely anxious? Your body may react physiologically. You may be short of breath, your heart may beat rapidly, you may feel all trembly, and you may feel like "I've got to get out of here!" You may try to relax, but are less effective in doing so. You may try to breathe deeply and find that the breath keeps catching in your throat. You may try to "shake the feeling" but you find that you can't. This becomes frightening and increases the anxiety even more. A vicious cycle quickly develops. Before long you feel completely out of control.

You also may be concerned about how others are perceiving you. They may see you as being out of control, or more importantly, your fear of them seeing you this way can become a self-fulfilling prophesy.

Which came first, the anxiety or the symptoms? It's really not important. What is more important is doing what is possible to reduce both.

IS FEAR GOOD OR BAD?

Believe it or not, fear is usually good! Now you're probably saying, "If I'm shaking with fear, how can it be good?" Fear mobilizes you. It "tells" you to prepare to attack the source of your fear. You react in a way that leads to action. In this regard, fear is similar to stress. It serves a necessary and critical purpose. In a way, it "protects" you.

Anxiety is bad if it is denied, or if it is so excessive that you can't do anything about it. If you face it and push past it, trying to resolve it, then fear is a positive emotion. It is only when the source of fear becomes overlooked, ignored, or denied that the consequences may be a problem. This is because the threat or danger is allowed to continue, and nothing (or not enough) is being done to control it.

HOW INTENSE ARE OUR REACTIONS?

Fear ranges in intensity from mild to severe. It is impossible to measure how much fear there is in anyone's life. It is unique and varies from person to person.

What determines how fearful you get? Usually the strength of the feared object, person, or event is important. Also, how close is it (wouldn't you be more afraid of getting an injection within the next thirty seconds, than if you were getting it in thirty days)? How vulnerable are you (do you hate injections, or are you just tired of feeling like a pincushion)? How successful are you in defending yourself (can you calmly accept the needle, or do you scream a lot)? These are some of the factors determining how you handle fear. Your own strength and the success of your defense mechanisms also play a role.

Randy, age thirty-one, was afraid to go to sleep at night. She was worried that she'd awaken in the middle of the night with palpitations. Since she had no symptoms before going to sleep, there was no reason to be afraid. But she didn't want to go to sleep. If Randy were stronger emotionally, she still might be concerned about palpitations, but she would not let it disturb her sleep. However, Randy wasn't strong. She was frightened. This fear kept her awake, she got less sleep, and she became more vulnerable to the very symptom she wanted to avoid!

People with MVP can be afraid of many things. Obviously, the more fears you have, the more these can interfere with your successful adjustment. Recognizing your fears and learning how to deal with them will help you live more happily and more comfortably. How? I was afraid you'd never ask!

HOW TO COPE WITH FEARS AND ANXIETIES

The first step in coping with your fears is to use the "pinpointing" technique discussed earlier. List all the things you're afraid of. Identify exactly what you are afraid of and exactly why you are afraid. Then think about what you can do to alleviate your fears. As you begin planning your strategies and gradually put your plan into operation, you'll continue to feel better and better.

Desensitize Yourself

A great technique used to conquer fear is called systematic desensitization. You learn to desensitize yourself, to make yourself less vulnerable to the source of your fear.

Here's how you can try it. Sit in a comfortable chair and relax. Then create a movie in your mind. Imagine what it is that makes you afraid. If you get tense, stop imagining it and relax. When you've calmed down, try imagining it again. The more you try to imagine your fear, the less it will bother you. Try it! It will give you a great feeling of relaxation and control. There are several library books that provide more information on systematic desensitization. Check them out.

An Anxious Thought

It was stated earlier that anxiety is a vague, uneasy feeling with an unknown source. So how can you cope with it by following the steps listed above? Well, if you try to pinpoint the source and are unable to, then you probably can't follow these specific steps. So what do you do? Use relaxation procedures. Work on changing your thinking. Even if you can't pinpoint a specific fear, these techniques will greatly help you to cope with general anxiety.

LET'S TALK ABOUT SPECIFICS

Remember, it is understandable for you to have many fears related to your condition. A problem arises, however, when you don't admit these fears. As a result, you don't do anything about resolving them. Just tell yourself that they can be resolved. Work on changing your thinking.

Initial Fears

When you were first diagnosed, many fearful questions probably came to mind. "What will the future be like? What will become of me? Will I die?" These are all typical questions of people who are diagnosed with many medical problems. As time has gone by since the diagnosis, in all probability some of these questions have been answered, and some of your initial qualms about having MVP have not materialized. But you're probably still afraid of some things. Let's discuss some of them.

Fear of Dying

When might you be most afraid of dying? Probably when you're in the middle of experiencing chest pain, or you feel like your heart is fluttering. Feeling the worst brings about fearing the worst! However, being afraid of dying is not going to help you feel better or live longer. If anything, it's only going to make you feel worse! Being afraid of dying, therefore, falls into the category of fears that you can do little or nothing about.

How do you attack this fear? Remember the facts. Chest pain with MVP is not the same as heart attack pain. Speak to your doctor. Remember that the field of medicine is constantly exploring new and improved treatment possibilities for individuals with mitral valve prolapse. So think positively. Others have had worse symptoms and still lived comfortably. Do you see how you must work on your thinking? If negative thoughts make you more afraid, then positive thoughts . . . !

When you're feeling better, with fewer symptoms, you're less likely to be afraid of dying. At that point you're more likely to be afraid of experiencing other symptoms.

By the way, as were mentioned before, some people who read medical information about MVP may read about a complication called sudden death. Sudden death is a very rare event in MVP. But, nevertheless, it can certainly be anxiety-provoking.

Although a very small number of individuals with MVP may die, this doesn't mean it's *because* of the MVP! There may not be any such conclusion about the cause of death. Any of a number of complications could have contributed to the death; these complications may not even be MVP-related! Work on your thinking so that this kind of fear doesn't overwhelm you.

Fear of Symptoms

Of course, sometimes even if you're following everything in your treatment program perfectly, you may still experience symptoms such as chest pain, shortness of breath, or extreme fatigue. You may be afraid of this. Can you defeat this fear? Yes. Try to plan what you're going to do when you experience any of these symptoms. For example, if you're afraid that fatigue will keep you from fulfilling your responsibilities, plan in advance what you'd do if there were things that needed to be done, and you temporarily couldn't do them because of exhaustion. Planning ahead can help reduce this fear.

Fear of Pain

Nobody likes pain. Pain is a very unpleasant part of MVP. You may be afraid of pain. This fear may be just as strong when you don't have pain, since you're afraid of it happening! If you do feel pain, you'll wonder when you're going to feel some relief. Each little twinge of pain may make you afraid of the worst, that your condition is not responding to treatment, or that additional problems exist or may develop.

What can you do about this fear? Try to accept the fact that some pain may occur from time to time, but medication can reduce its intensity (as well as its frequency). Further suggestions will be offered in the chapter on Pain. Realize that each pain "cycle" will eventually stop or at least ease up. It won't last forever.

Fear of Medication and Possible Side Effects

You may be nervous about any medications that you've been told to take, even though you need them. You may be afraid of any potential damage to your body. Just keep reminding yourself that if your doctor prescribed medication for you, then there must be a reason. Your physician is aware of any possible side effects. But as long as the advantages of the medication outweigh the side effects, medication will still be prescribed.

Fear of "What Next?"

What will happen next? You can't be sure. Will there be an increase in the amount of pain? Will you develop new symptoms? Will your heart be damaged because of any added strain placed on it? Will you develop any side effects from your medication? Fear of "what next?" includes being afraid of new symptoms, or the return of old ones.

Everyone wonders what's in store for the future. But because of the unpleasantness of what you've experienced, you may be afraid of the future, rather than merely curious. What can you do? Unless you own a crystal ball, you can't foresee what will happen in the future. So take life one day at a time. What will be, will be. (What a great name for a song!) Just tell yourself that you'll handle any problems as they occur. As long as you're doing what you have to in order to take care of yourself, there's nothing else you can do anyway.

Fear of Not Being Believed

Are you in pain? Are you "wiped out" from fatigue? Do you find it hard to constantly let other people know how you feel? Maybe you're afraid that others just won't believe you. "I can't believe that anybody would experience as much as you do with mitral valve prolapse," you're afraid they're thinking. You know what you're feeling, but it's frightening to think that other people just will not understand. You don't want to be labeled a hypochondriac! What to do? Talk to the nonbelievers. Share reading material with them. Try to explain MVP as best as you can. You've then done all you can. You can't crawl into someone else's head and change beliefs.

Fear of Others' Reactions

Are you afraid that other people will shy away from you because of MVP? You may fear rejection if you can't socialize the way you'd like to be able to. Others may feel you can't keep up with them. But don't try, because pushing yourself can be a painful way to maintain a friendship.

Unfortunately, some people can be cold and unfeeling. Who needs those kinds of friends anyway? Other friends will accept you under any circumstances. Enjoy them. But since you can't change the way some people feel, try not to be as concerned with their reactions. Instead, be more attentive to your own needs and feelings.

Other fears in this category can be even more frightening. "What if my spouse leaves me? What if all my friends stay away from me?" Isolation can be a horrible thought. If it's not happening now, you may be afraid of it happening in the future. You may be afraid that none of your friends will remain "in your corner." To reduce the chances of such rejection, you may hesitate to make plans with friends or family. This would only add to your feeling of isolation.

Consider your thoughts, but be realistic. Remember that a change in a social relationship can occur for any reason, not just because of MVP! If you feel that your relationship is in jeopardy, try to figure out what this might be, and see what you can do to help ("put all your cards on the table," discuss problems, even get counseling, if need be). But you can do only so much. If that doesn't work, even though the outcome may upset you, at least you know you've tried.

Fear of Overdoing/Underdoing

You may not know how much you should do. You may be afraid of doing too much, but you may feel guilty about doing too little! How do you conquer this? Get advice from experts. You need professional advice in coming up with the best "mix" of rest and exercise. And you'll need to know which, if any, activities may be too strenuous for you. Even your doctor may not have specific answers. You may be told that the answers will become apparent only through trial-and-error. You can learn only through experience. So what should you do? Pace yourself. Change your level of activity gradually. Then tell yourself, as with so many other fears, that you're doing the best you can.

Fear of Employment Problems

You may be concerned about whether or not you'll be able to keep your job. You may want to work, but fear that you won't be able to. Your employer may be understanding at first, but you worry about how long this will continue. And, of course, you may be afraid of all the money problems that might result if you can't work. Can you do much to change the nature of this fear? You can evaluate your vocational skills and make sure you have a job that you can handle. Other than this, you'll have to live with this fear, and just hope for the best. If there's a problem, you'll cope. Being afraid won't help.

Fear of Loss of Income

Any medical problem leads to greater financial obligations. Because of this, your need for money will be greater, too! If you can't work, this pressure is even greater. Medical bills have to be paid. You can't depend on insurance plans, since they don't always provide enough coverage. In addition, many insurance plans require you to pay the doctor first and then get reimbursed. Doctors' fees can be quite high, and if the money is not coming in. . . . What can you do? Talk to people. See what other people do. Maybe you'll get some ideas that will help you to conquer this fear. And remember, you'll work it out. When was the last time that you read of someone being thrown out on the street, penniless, because of MVP?

Fear of Treatment Troubles

What if you've had problems with your treatment? It seems like you've experienced unpleasant side effects with every medication you've tried. None of the therapies you've tried has done any good. You just can't get into an exercise routine. You begin to fear that nothing is really going to make a difference. Yes, there are some people who have more difficulty than others adapting to a treatment program. And it's possible you may not benefit as much as you (or your doctor, family, therapists, friends, etc.) would like.

Hang in there. New medications and techniques are being developed all the time. And, who knows? More trial-and-error may just come up with a solution. Giving up just makes you more tense and uncomfortable, anyway. So keep trying. Remember: A positive mental attitude is one of the cornerstones of your treatment program. So by working on this, you know you're accomplishing something.

Fear of Children Having MVP

The thought of your children going through what you are may be so frightening that you may not want to have children. But even if you already have a family, you may be panicky. You don't want to live in constant fear of your child developing the same symptoms.

Learn the facts. Yes, it's possible for your children to develop MVP, but there are no guarantees that it will happen. And even if they do have the structural valve problem, that doesn't mean they'll experience the symptoms of MVP Syndrome. But even if they do experience any other symptoms, they can learn to deal with them just as you are. Who's to say that the future can't look bright anyway? Lots of buts, right? But (yes, one more) keep thinking positively.

If your child is diagnosed with MVP, it need not be the end of the world. It's not your fault. Your child still "wanted" to be born and to be alive. Maybe you'll be able to help one another adjust. But don't resign yourself to the fact that your child is destined to have mitral valve prolapse until a diagnosis is made (if ever). Otherwise, you're blowing your fear all out of proportion. Remember, treatment is improving and will likely be even better as your children grow up than it is now. A diagnosis of mitral valve prolapse is not a disaster.

Fear of Fear

This section also might have been called "Fear of Anxiety," or " Fear of Panic Attacks," or any of a number of other possibilities. What they all mean, though, is that many people who are uncomfortable being anxious or experiencing fear become frightened of experiencing these reactions again. These are called secondary anxiety reactions, meaning that you're not afraid of a specific object, person, or situation as much as you're anxious about being anxious!

What to do? Start by using relaxation techniques. Then tell yourself that you'll work on dealing with any situation (or feeling) as it occurs, rather than worrying about what might or might not ever happen. Reread the information in this chapter and in the next chapter on Panic. And, if necessary, work with a supportive professional to help you deal with this.

Fear of Not Coping

You may feel that you're barely handling having mitral valve prolapse. You may think that any new problem that comes along will be enough to push you over the edge. Fear of falling apart can easily lead to panic: an out-of-control kind of feeling that will make you fall apart.

Get a hold of yourself. Pinpoint those particular things you're having difficulty with, and get help in dealing with them. Don't wait. Don't project a false sense of bravado that you can and must handle everything yourself. If you feel yourself near the edge, get someone to help you to steady yourself. Talk it over with someone. Once you share your feelings and fears with someone, you may see things a little more clearly. You may be able to deal with problems with greater strength, knowing that you're not alone. Once you're back in control, this fear will disappear.

A FEARLESS SUMMARY

Although many different fears have been discussed in this chapter, we probably have not covered all of the ones you have experienced. In addition, the coping suggestions offered certainly do not include all possible ways of dealing with fear. So what should you do?

You're working on recognizing your fears, right? For some of them, you're modifying your behavior. For others, you're modifying your thinking. Soon you will feel more in control. As this happens, you'll notice your fears begin to diminish. That doesn't mean that they'll all go away. But as you work on them and feel more in control, they'll at least lessen in intensity. You'll feel better knowing that you can do something about some of them and that you're capable of handling them.

9

Panic

When fear or anxiety increases beyond the "typical" level, we get what is unpleasantly known as panic. Panic is considered to be an extreme form of anxiety. Research suggests that approximately 5 percent of the general population suffers from panic disorders. It is also estimated that 80 percent of those with panic disorders are women. Panic attacks are an unfortunate symptom for some people with MVP.

Panic may strike suddenly and without warning. Occasionally, there may not even appear to be a specific trigger. Or, the trigger may be perfectly clear, but still nothing can be done to prevent the panic attack.

As you learned in the last chapter, although there are times that anxiety can be beneficial to an individual, panic is usually at such an intense level that there are few if any, benefits to the experience. So let's discuss more about panic, and what can be done about it.

WHAT DO PANIC ATTACKS FEEL LIKE?

When panic attacks occur, they can be devastating! You feel like you are losing control, and you're petrified about what's going to happen next. These feelings are usually overwhelming. Considering how powerful these feelings are, it's not surprising that it is practically impossible, at this time, to identify what it is that triggered the attack!

SYMPTOMS OF PANIC ATTACKS

The physical symptoms that are most common in a panic attack are palpitations, increased heart rate and blood flow, pounding heart, chest pain, sweating, dizziness, shortness of breath, imbalance, disoriented feelings, a feeling of suffocation, rubbery legs, flushing, numbness, nausea, a lump in the throat, and light-headedness. (Even this sounds frightening!)

But the list doesn't end there. There are also psychological symptoms, including emotional feelings of going crazy, fear of dying, fear of losing control, a feeling of impending doom, and an extreme desire to escape from the given situation. Wonderful, right? So, some of the symptoms are psychological, but a good number of them are physiological. The physiological components are triggered by sudden bursts of adrenaline, which normally is released in bodies under stress. This stress response has also been called the "fight or flight" syndrome. (You'll read more about this in the chapter on Stress.)

WHY IS IT SO HARD TO STOP A PANIC ATTACK?

If you are experiencing a panic attack, it may be very difficult for you to view the situation rationally and realize that there is nothing to be afraid of. Rather, you may be unable to think objectively at all, and your emotions will take over. The fear can then become more and more intense.

The more you feel unable to control panic attacks, the more often they may occur. In part, this may be because it will take less stress to trigger a panic attack, since you feel out of control to begin with.

There are times that panic attacks can be of very short duration. They may only last for a few minutes or so and then they pass. There are other times, though, when panic attacks last up to an hour or more. That can be devastating!

Because of the desire to do something to stop panic attacks, they may lead to the onset of phobias. Why? Phobias, irrational fears of a situation or object, actually start as avoidance behavior. You may start associating the discomfort of panic attacks with whatever situations you were in at the time that the attacks began. You'll then try to avoid these situations more and more, and finally become phobic in your intense need to avoid those situations.

WHAT CAUSES PANIC ATTACKS?

Much research has focused on possible biochemical causes for panic attacks. Many experts in the field believe that panic does have, to at least some degree, a biochemical basis. For example, some researchers suggest that panic attacks in women are more common just prior to menstruation. It may be that the change in the level of progesterone, a female hormone, can trigger the attack.

Psychological Causes

Although we have been discussing the biochemical basis of panic attacks, psychological factors are certainly involved as well. In some cases, individuals who experience panic attacks have experienced some kind of stress just prior to the onset of the attack. Yes, it is true that the stress may only be mild. But if the person is especially vulnerable, it need not be more than a mild stressor to trigger the physiological response that leads to a panic attack.

So yes, psychological factors may be involved. But it is important to remember that psychological factors, by themselves, usually do not trigger the extreme reaction that we know as panic attacks. Usually, the combination of the stressor and the internal physiological response is what creates a panic attack.

Panic Attacks and MVP

Although there have been many people with MVP who have experienced panic attacks, research has still not proven either that panic attacks cause MVP, or that MVP causes panic attacks. What does this mean? The most logical conclusion drawn by many scientists is that MVP and panic attacks may simply be occurring at the same time.

Are there any possible explanations for these "coincidences"? Why is it that some individuals with MVP may have a greater chance of having panic attacks? This may be because of the connection between MVP and the autonomic nervous system, as well as possible hormonal involvement. Remember, in MVP, you may already be experiencing an imbalance in your autonomic nervous system. As a result, if you experience something stressful, such as an unpleasant event or a frightening encounter, the imbalance in your autonomic nervous system may become even more pronounced. The shortness of breath, the experiencing of chest pain, or a rapid heartbeat, may also become more pronounced because of the imbalance in the autonomic nervous system. Guess what? That can cause even more of an anxious or panicky response.

Certain chemicals may increase your susceptibility to panic attacks. Drugs such as cocaine or marijuana may contribute to panic attack symptoms. Fatigue due to a medical problem may make you more vulnerable to panic because your defense system may be too low to begin with. Caffeine may make you more susceptible to panic attacks. (This is one of the reasons that many professionals suggest a decrease of caffeine consumption if you have experienced panic attacks, whether or not you have MVP.)

So let's summarize what we know. MVP and panic attacks may both have a basis in the autonomic nervous system. They both require treatment so that they don't exacerbate each other. Individuals experiencing both disorders experience a number of similar symptoms, such as chest pain, fatigue, palpitations, dizziness, and light-headedness. Although it seems that specific treatment for MVP will not necessarily have a bearing on panic, and specific treatment for panic will not necessarily have a bearing on MVP, you should still look to be more comfortable and deal better with whatever is affecting you!

TREATMENT FOR PANIC

Much of the treatment for panic initially involves the same approach as the techniques you read about in the previous chapter. You'll want to try to pinpoint what may be triggering your panic attack and see if you can change, or even eliminate, these triggers. (If you can't pinpoint them at the time of the attack, at least try to think about them when you have calmed down!) You'll want to use relaxation techniques to increase your feelings of being in control. You'll want to work on your thinking to restructure any negative thoughts that may be contributing to or exacerbating the panic.

In some cases, using these techniques can bring about a sufficient degree of control over panic. If more panic attacks continue to occur, however, there are three other components of treatment.

Medication

The first component is medication. Because there is a biological component to panic, it may be necessary to treat this with panic medication. The medications used are designed to block whatever is biochemically contributing to the onset or exacerbation of panic.

It is very important that the person's autonomic nervous system be stabilized. This is done to try to keep any potential initiating triggers or stressors from creating the extreme kind of physiological responses that are most common in panic attacks.

There are three categories of medications that can be helpful in dealing with panic attacks: benzodiazapines, tricyclic antidepressants, and the amino oxidase inhibitors (MAO inhibitors). More information on the many medications that can be helpful in treating panic attacks will be provided in the chapter on medications. However, keep in mind that although a medication may be beneficial in dealing with panic attacks, it may not be necessarily indicated in patients who have MVP.

Behavior Therapy

Second, because panic can lead to additional anxieties and phobias, these phobias must be treated psychologically with behavior therapy. Techniques such as systematic desensitization, discussed in the previous chapter, can be very effective in reducing phobias.

Psychotherapy

Third, any psychosocial stressors or complicating events should be handled with psychotherapy. Because panic attacks can be so extreme, they often require professional intervention. This is especially true if they occur often. Don't feel "weak" if you decide to consult with a professional. After all, your goal is to feel better, right? If you have difficulty resolving some of these problems yourself, isn't it good to know that there are experts you can work with who can help you regain control?

10

Anger

Annie, age thirty-one, was fed up with chest pain. She was tired of being told she was imagining things, and was frustrated that nothing her doctor did would diminish the pain. Practically anyone who went near her received an earful of comments you wouldn't want Mother to hear! Everyone was a victim of this verbal assault, from her doctor to her family. Was Annie angry? You bet your eardrums she was!

In general, people with any chronic medical problem may be angry. Because anger results in the build-up of physical energy that needs to be released, it is important for you to learn how to cope with anger.

WHAT IS ANGER?

When you have a desire or goal in mind and something interferes with your achieving it, this can be very frustrating. A feeling of tension and hostility may result. This is what we refer to as anger.

THREE TYPES OF ANGER

It can be helpful to discuss three different ways of experiencing anger. Rage is the expression of violent, uncontrolled anger. If Annie was feeling upset about her condition, and a "friend" told her that she wouldn't be so uncomfortable if she didn't get so upset all the time, you can imagine how angry she might be. Her anger might even lead her to say or do things that would certainly not enhance the prospects of a long-lasting, warm relationship with this person!

Rage is probably the most intense anger you can experience. It is an outward expression of anger, because there is noticeable evidence of a visible explosion. Rage can be a destructive release of the intense physical energy that builds up.

A second type of anger is resentment. This is the feeling of anger that is usually kept inside. What if Annie listened to her friend's well-meaning comments, smiled and said nothing, but was seething inside? Resentment is a growing, smoldering feeling of anger directed toward a person or an object. However, it is often kept bottled up. It tends to sit uncomfortably within you, and can create even more physiological and psychological damage.

The third type of anger is indignation. Indignation is considered the more appropriate, positive type of anger. It is released in a more controlled way. If Annie had responded to the comments by stating that she appreciated her friend's concern, but would prefer no advice at this point or she might scream, this might have been a more appropriate response.

Obviously, these three types of anger can occur in combination, or in different ways. However, understanding the different ways of experiencing anger can help you to cope with it more effectively.

CAUSES OF ANGER

Obviously, there are lots of things that can make you angry. You may get angry if you have to wait for your doctor to see you. You may get angry if you feel your family is not helping you enough. You may get angry if you have to cancel plans at the last minute.

Insults from other people, aside from everyday frustrations, can cause anger. "If you got more sleep at night, you wouldn't have those problems." This is not the kind of comment that may make you feel friendly! If you feel that someone is taking advantage of you, or you feel forced to do something that you do not want to do, anger may result. Your friend says, "I have this party next Saturday. You have such good taste in clothes, please come with me to pick out a dress. We'll only go to seven or eight stores." If you do not have the ability or confidence to say "no" when friends ask for a favor, this can create feelings of anger, especially when combined with the fact that you may feel too fatigued to go.

In addition to the causes of anger mentioned above, there is one more. How about mitral valve prolapse as a cause of anger? Aren't you angry about this? There may not be any specific reason you can point to. Or you might be able to list dozens of reasons. But being aware of this is important, because you must be aware of the anger to help yourself deal with it. Unfortunately, resolving your anger won't make MVP go away. Nor should you say that you'll stop being angry only when your condition is a thing of the past. Neither attitude will help you. As we go on, we will be discussing ways of reducing anger and feeling better.

Does Your Mind Make You Angry?

It is important to realize that anger exists uniquely in the mind of each angry individual. This anger is a direct result of your thoughts, rather than events. The event by itself does not make you angry. Rather, it leads to your interpretation of the event, the way you think or feel about it. That's what can make you angry! This is a very important point, one that will be discussed in much more detail a little bit later in the section "Dealing With Anger." Stay tuned . . .

ANGER AND YOUR BODY

When you are angry, a number of physiological responses occur in your body. Breathing becomes more rapid, blood pressure increases (you may feel like your blood is "boiling"), and your heart may begin to pound. Your face may get "hot," and your muscles become tense. You may feel stronger when angry. The more intense the anger is, the greater this feeling of power. I'm sure you can remember a time when you were so angry that you felt you had superhuman strength.

Anger is a form of energy. The more physical energy that builds up in the body due to anger, the more necessary it becomes for you to release it. This energy cannot be destroyed. So if it is not released in some constructive manner, it will eventually come out in another, less desirable way.

Imagine the energy from anger as a stick of dynamite about to explode. If you get rid of it, it will explode away from you. It may cause some damage, but it will not hurt you inside as much as if you swallowed the dynamite to keep others from being hurt. Obviously, the ideal solution is not to throw the stick of dynamite, and not to swallow it, but (are you ready for this?) to try to defuse the dynamite! More about defusing soon.

Usually, extreme anger passes quickly. If, however, the anger lasts for a long period of time, it can have physically damaging effects on the body. You've all heard about some of the physical problems that can result from holding in anger: for example, ulcers, hypertension, headaches. Anger can also cause a stress response that may exacerbate your medical condition. It's just not good for your body.

When anger becomes extreme or turns into rage, you may feel like exploding. You may feel that unless you are able to punch, kick, or hit something and get rid of the anger in some way, you will lose control. Hopefully, this angry energy can be released without causing damage to another person, property, or yourself. If, when you finally calm down, you find that you have done something destructive, you may get angry with yourself all over again. Or you may experience another negative emotion, such as guilt.

ANGER AND YOUR MIND

Anger is usually experienced as a very unpleasant feeling. However, this unpleasant feeling may exist along with a more pleasant feeling of power or strength. Frequently, the unpleasantness of anger is related to its consequences—knowing what you do when you are angry, and not being happy about it. If you lose control when you're angry, you'll probably even be afraid of it, and of what you might do next time!

DIFFERENT REACTIONS TO ANGER

Maureen, a twenty-eight-year-old teacher, was having a hard time with her husband. He was trying to show concern for his wife by not letting her do any housework. But, surprisingly, she wanted to clean the house because she believed she felt well enough to do it. His resistance was so persistent, and he was so "saccharin sweet," that Maureen felt it was too much. She wanted to be treated like an adult, able to determine when she could be active. But her husband just wouldn't let up. She was running out of patience. Let's see how this situation might be experienced in different ways.

The "Ignore" Approach

Because you feel like you may completely lose control, or feel over-whelmed by the intensity of your anger, you may try to do whatever you can to avoid the experience. This could include pushing thoughts out of your mind, even when you realize you are getting angry. Maureen might try to get involved in different activities while her husband cleans the house, and try to ignore the fact that she feels he is being condescending. Or she might try to agree with everything that he says. Although this might be upsetting, it might at least be temporarily effective in helping her to ignore the smothering. In the long run, however, you can see that this is not the best way to deal with anger.

The "Action" Approach

Maureen might know that she's not happy being angry and that she should speak to her husband to try to get him to understand more about her emotional needs and how she'd like him to treat her. Hopefully, a better understanding can be reached, but at least Maureen knows that she's doing something about her feelings.

In this case, you might see anger as a necessary part of life, despite its unpleasantness. You know that there will be times when you'll be angry, whether you like it or not. You'll just have to deal with it as best you can.

The "Power" Approach

Maybe you enjoy the flow of energy and strength that comes from being angry. You may find that this is when you are best able to assert yourself to accomplish something. Here, Maureen knows that if she is smothered once too often she will explode, and she loves the feeling of power that this anger gives her. She is almost looking forward to the chance to say, "Honey, if you treat me that way once more, I'll take this vacuum cleaner and . . . !" That would wipe the smile off hubby's face!

If you enjoy this feeling, it's possible that you may even provoke situations to make yourself angry! An example of this would be professional football players or boxers, who psyche themselves up before a confrontation with an opponent. For them, becoming as angry as possible is the best preparation for a successful performance.

Your own reaction to anger is unique. It may also change from time to time. There may be times when you accept anger and almost value it as a motivator to accomplish something. At other times you may attempt to push this anger away. Maureen might enjoy expressing her anger. But if she didn't want to cause problems with or hurt her husband, or upset the rest of the family, she might realize that it would be better to have a calm discussion with him than to shatter his eardrums with her explosion.

IS ANGER GOOD OR BAD?

How can anger possibly be good? Many people feel that nothing constructive can be gained from it. "Avoid anger at all costs," they say, "because nothing good comes from it. . . . Anger will get you into trouble, so don't let it happen." This is true, but only if you don't deal with the anger properly. Anger can be dangerous if it is kept inside. Remember that stick of dynamite? What an explosive example! If anger is released in destructive ways, it can cause problems in relationships (to say the least!). It can create physical problems as well, and can certainly aggravate your MVP-related problems. Does this mean that anger can make your condition worse? Well, what if you're so angry with somebody or something that you decide not to take proper care of yourself? For example, you don't take your medication properly, taking too much or too little, almost like you're sticking your tongue out at the world. Or what if being angry with someone or something causes you to do more than you should be doing. "I'll show them," you say. Having mitral valve prolapse, you know that you don't want to wear yourself down.

What if you're angry with someone who cares about you, and is normally supportive of you in dealing with MVP? That person, if upset by your anger, may be less willing to help you. This may, in turn, make you feel even worse. So if you want your anger to be good instead of bad, try to turn it into something that can be helpful rather than harmful to you.

Anger can be constructive. It can mobilize your efforts and make you stronger to deal with an anger-provoking situation. Believe it or not, you might even handle a situation more successfully than you would if you weren't angry!

Anger can give you a feeling of power or strength, of confidence or assertiveness. But don't get me wrong. I'm not saying that you should slam your finger with a hammer, or tell someone to punch you, in order to get yourself angry enough to solve all of your problems! What I am saying is that anger can be positive, and, if used correctly, can help you to solve problems.

Anger has two main benefits. First, it is an indicator that something is wrong. Something must be creating this angry feeling—something that needs attention. Second, anger can motivate you to deal more actively with life's problems. You can become so emotionally charged that it will have a positive effect on your life.

In order for anger to be helpful, there are some very important things to keep in mind. First, don't let yourself become overwhelmed by the anger. Once that happens it is much harder to do what you have to do. Second, don't be afraid of your anger. If you do fear it, you probably won't be able to release it properly. More than likely, it will come out in unhealthy ways, or you'll bottle it up inside. Third, be sure that the way you handle your anger is socially acceptable. Maureen might get a kick out of knocking out her husband's teeth, but would the police (or the dentist) approve? Try to be flexible enough to recognize an appropriate way of releasing your anger.

DEALING WITH ANGER

You've already begun to realize that anger can be constructive. Hopefully, the information you've read so far has been encouraging. But what else can actually be done?

Because anger is such a complex emotion, and because so many things can lead to feelings of anger, there are no simple answers. Sorry about that! Does that mean that there is nothing that anybody can do about anger? No. Some things can be done to reduce the feelings of anger and allow them to be handled more efficiently, comfortably, and safely.

Step One: Admit That You're Angry

The first step in dealing with anger is to recognize that you're angry in the first place. As simple as this may sound, many people cannot even admit when they're angry. They may try to deny it, or rationalize their feelings or behaviors using other explanations.

Do you feel that being angry is a sign of weakness? If so, since you don't want to feel weak, you may not even admit that you're angry. You may feel that there is no appropriate reason to be angry, so you're acting in a childish way. But as with anything else, in order to try to change something, you've first got to admit that it exists.

How can you tell that you're angry if you're not sure? (Yes, there are some people who are not sure.) If you feel very tense (jumping at the sound of the telephone), or if you find yourself reacting impulsively (slamming down the phone when you get a wrong number and storming out of the house) or with hostility (cursing at your neighbor for leaving a smidgen of garbage on your lawn), chances are that you're angry. Until you recognize that you are angry, you cannot do anything constructive about it.

Step Two: Where Does Your Anger Come From?

The second step in dealing with anger is trying to identify its source. Where does it come from? What is contributing to it? What events have led to these feelings of anger? Why do you want to break all the furniture? For one thing, your condition may lead to anger. You may feel anger toward your physician, whether justified or not. You may be angry because you have to change your diet. You may be angry because you feel so out of control.

In some cases, the events leading to anger may be quite obvious. In other cases, however, the source of anger may be vague and unclear. It may be hard to pinpoint what is causing it. At such times, you should try to probe even more deeply to come up with possible causes of your anger.

Take, for example, the case of Suzanne, a forty-seven-year-old homemaker. She was awakened one bright, cheerful morning to hear birds singing right outside her bedroom. Instead of feeling happy and carefree, she felt angry. She had just awakened, but she felt angry. Initially, she was unable to figure out why, on such a beautiful day, she might feel angry. But finally, after giving the matter a lot of thought, she realized that because it was sunny and bright out, her detested cousins were going to come from out of town to visit, and she would feel obligated to entertain them, something that she did not wish to do. Remember: Being able to identify the source of anger is very important in being able to deal with it.

Of course, much of this anger is irrational. But, like other emotional reactions, it must be worked through. It cannot just be pushed away. Simply telling yourself, "Don't be angry," is not enough. You must learn to channel it more effectively.

Guilt can sometimes confuse you if you are trying to identify the source of anger. Margaret was a thirty-three-year-old mother of three. She woke up one morning, went downstairs and found her kitchen a disaster area. Taking care of the kitchen was a responsibility that she had given to her children, because she was simply physically unable to handle it. She found herself screaming at them for not fulfilling their responsibilities. In actuality, however, her anger may have been a reflection, not of hostility toward her children, but of guilt about her own inability to handle her kitchen responsibilities.

Step Three: Why Are You Angry?

It is now necessary to explain to yourself why you are angry. In Margaret's case, she could explain her anger by her inability to do what she wanted to do. Margaret wanted to be able to fulfill her responsibilities as a mother and housewife. She felt that taking care of the kitchen was included in this. Because she was unable to do so, she felt angry.

Why is this step important? Mainly, to decide whether or not the anger that you are feeling is realistic. Analyze your reasons for being angry. If you recognize that your reasons are not realistic, this alone can help you to deal with these feelings of anger. If, on the other hand, you can objectively say that your feelings of anger are realistic, then the next step is to decide how you are going to deal with them properly.

How do you deal with them properly? You have already begun! By working through the first three steps, you have received information that will be very helpful in your efforts to deal with your anger.

THOUGHTS CAN MAKE YOU ANGRY

In the past, it was falsely believed that there were only two possible ways to deal with anger: to keep it inside, or to let it out.

But what about a third possibility? Remember before when we talked about defusing that stick of dynamite? Our anger is a result of the way we think! In our minds, we are actually interpreting those events that lead to anger. If we can change the way we interpret events and reorganize our thinking patterns, is it possible to stop creating the anger that we feel? Of course! We can learn to control our thoughts before they make us angry, regardless of what the events were.

Ask yourself this question: If something happened that made you angry, would everybody in the world be angry because of it? No. The reason you are angry is that this is the way *you* think about, or interpret, the event. Other people may not be angry because they did not interpret the event in a way that made them so. For example, let's say you've made a doctor's appointment. Ten minutes before you were ready to leave, the receptionist called to cancel, saying she'd reschedule the appointment at another time. You might be furious, because you felt you should have received more notice, and because you really wanted to be seen. How aggravating!! But others might not interpret it that way, and might not get the least bit angry. So if we can learn to interpret events in a more positive, constructive, and calm manner, we can reduce feelings of anger. We wouldn't have to decide whether we wanted to let anger out or keep it inside because, by controlling our thoughts, anger would not even exist most of the time.

You've already completed one of the first steps in reorganizing your thoughts to prevent anger. You've learned that anger can be good and constructive. It can help you to solve problems, and you don't have to be afraid of it. Just becoming aware of its positive elements can help you to be less afraid of anger. This can help you to deal with the thoughts that may make you angry.

Good Angry Thoughts Vs. Bad Angry Thoughts

Writing down what you think is making you angry can be very helpful. Good angry thoughts can move you to positive, constructive action. You might want to plan your strategies for resolving the problem. On the other hand, many of your thoughts may include so much anger, and be so destructive, that you feel like banging your head against the wall. Be honest when writing down your thoughts, regardless of how violent or profane they may be! Such rich, colorful language can be helpful in getting your feelings out and down on paper. This will ultimately help you to control your anger. Try to look at these thoughts more objectively, the way someone else might look at them. Attempt to bring them down to a more manageable level.

Mental Movies

An interesting technique that can be helpful in controlling anger is imagery, or "watching movies in your mind." When you become angry, you frequently have all kinds of pictures in your head of what is making you angry and what you'd like to do to deal with it. These movies can be very helpful.

For example, imagine that you are very, very tired. Your friend calls to tell you that her car has broken down. Could you please pick up her dry-cleaning? When you tell her that you are too tired to go, she says something about how she can never depend on you for anything. This is a friend? You are furious. At that moment, imagine all the abusive things that you would like to say to her, and imagine the shocked expression on her face. If you ask her to hold on for a moment, and close your eyes and imagine this as if you were actually doing it, you'll probably be able to complete the phone call without destroying a friendship. You may even smile or laugh as you think about the scenes that are playing through your mind. More about imagery in the chapter "Pain."

Nora was quite fed up with her son, Pesty Pete. Whenever she asked for his help with normal household chores, his answers were fresh and abusive. Just before she was about to give him a haircut with a meat cleaver, she remembered the mental movie technique. She imagined herself strangling him—his eyeballs popping and gurgling sounds coming from his throat. This helped to get rid of the intense, angry feelings that were making her crazy, and allowed her to deal with Pete more constructively. (No, she's not in jail.)

The Big Red Stop Sign

Another technique that can help you to control anger is referred to as "thought stopping." Remember: It is the thoughts in your mind that are making you angry. These are the thoughts you have when you interpret an event. When you find that angry thoughts have come into your head, picture a big red stop sign. Seeing that picture in your mind will serve as a momentary distraction. Then concentrate on something you enjoy. This can be a peaceful, relaxing scene, a type of food that you like to eat, an activity that you enjoy, or a movie or television program. Whatever you choose, you will divert your thinking, and have a better chance of dissipating your anger. You also could participate in a pleasant distracting activity, such as reading a book, taking a walk, or calling a friend, which also can help you to feel less angry.

Change Your Requirements

People often get angry when they want certain things to occur in certain ways. When your specific requirements are not met, you may feel angry. Trying to modify your requirements can help you to cope with anger.

Let's say that you're not feeling well and you decide to call your doctor. The answering service tells you that he is not in the office and that you should get a return call within a half-hour. After forty-five minutes, when he has still not returned your call, you are fuming. Why? Because your requirement of a call-back within thirty minutes has not been met. What to do? Revise your requirement. Tell yourself that you would have liked a call within thirty minutes, but your doctor may be tied up on another case, or in transit, or unable to get to a phone. You'll be satisfied if you get a call at his earliest convenience. By modifying the requirement, you can feel less angry.

Another way to benefit from this technique is to write down those thoughts indicating what your requirements are. Then try to write down new, more flexible desires. This will make you feel better.

Put Yourself in Their Shoes

One of the best ways of dealing with anger toward somebody else is to try to understand exactly what that person is feeling: what the person wants, or why the person is saying what he or she is saying. This will make you more aware of why somebody else is behaving or talking the way he or she is, and you will be better able to deal with it constructively. This also will help you to understand what the other person will feel if he or she is the target of your abusive release of anger.

LET IT OUT LESS EXPLOSIVELY

We have discussed a number of ways to control your thinking and improve your ability to interpret events in ways that will not allow anger to develop. But what if this doesn't always work? What if there are times when you remain as angry as you were before? What can be done to deal with anger constructively when it already exists?

Talk. Don't Bite.

Obviously, it is much more desirable to have a constructive discussion over an issue than an angry exchange of heated words that accomplishes nothing. In most cases, anger can arise if you have a conflict or problem with another person. Therefore, it can really be helpful to improve your ability to get your point across constructively. You are trying to negotiate a better resolution to a problem that may exist between you and somebody else. A heated argument, or "fighting fire with fire," is not the answer. Instead, you want to fight the fire by dousing it—reducing the heatedness of the argument. How? Try complimenting the person or looking for the positive things in what that person is saying to you. Yes, do this even if you're angry. This works in two ways. One, it will probably surprise the person. Two, you'll be focusing on words or thoughts that are more constructive, rather than letting yourself get angry because of what's being said. Then calmly restate your feelings.

Let's take the previous example where you are upset at your friend's demands to pick up the dry-cleaning. Instead of blowing up at her and telling her that she is so inconsiderate and just doesn't understand, tell her she's right in calling you. You're glad she thought of you. But then let her know that as much as you would like to do this favor for her, you don't even have the strength to get dressed. Keep looking for something positive to respond to regardless of what she says, and calmly continue to indicate that you don't feel well. Eventually you'll get the point across. Although she may not be too happy about it (she may even get angry), you will have been able to resolve a problem in a constructive way, with much less anger.

How About Physical Activity?

In general, one of the best outlets for releasing angry energy is physical activity. But what if, because of mitral valve prolapse, this outlet is not as available as you'd like? Besides being angry about something else, it can be frustrating if having mitral valve prolapse requires you to reduce your physical activity. Because you may be prone to fatigue and have less energy, this outlet may not be readily usable. But there is a solution. Some people find that physical energy from anger can be released by watching things! For example, by watching a sporting event, you aren't releasing energy through participation in the sport, but you may still be able to "get into it" and reduce your anger that way. Or try watching a particularly violent or emotionally draining movie. You can become so totally absorbed that the energy building up from anger is released through worry, fear, or excitement. A movie or book that allows you to identify with the characters, or where the characters allow release of anger, can be beneficial as well.

A common and very effective outlet for anger, especially among children, is crying. I'm sure you've heard of the therapeutic effects of a good cry. However, this technique is not for everyone. People who can be more open in expressing their emotions may be better able to benefit from this outlet.

Some people like to count to ten when angry. This can distract you from what is making you angry, giving you a chance to calm down and think about it more constructively. Try counting to one thousand, if necessary!

LET US REVIEW

It is very important to remember that events alone do not make you angry. It is your thoughts, your interpretations of these events, that lead to anger. Even if something really terrible happens, it is the meaning that you give to this particular event that makes you angry. It is the way you think about this terrible event that creates your anger. Since your thinking makes you angry, you are responsible for feeling this way. Therefore, you can be just as responsible for changing your thinking to help yourself cope with anger, or at least reducing it to a more manageable level.

The best way to handle anger is probably to be in control enough so that it doesn't build up in the first place. But if it does, remember that if anger is channeled and used constructively, it does have its benefits. Uncontrolled anger can be an unpleasant, negative, destructive emotion. Your efforts are best spent in trying to figure out how to reorganize your thinking so that it doesn't get out of hand.

11

Guilt

Have you ever felt guilty? Many individuals with MVP say that they have. Guilt is a very unpleasant emotion. Take the case of Nell, a twenty-eight-year-old mother of three. She was very unhappy because one of her favorite activities was playing tennis with her husband. Now, because of MVP, her doctor suggested she try more subdued activities for awhile. She felt guilty that she was not being the tennis player she knew her husband wanted. So having mitral valve prolapse made her feel guilty that she was being a bad wife. Hard to cope? You bet! Let's take a look at what leads to guilty feelings.

THE TWO COMPONENTS OF GUILT

Feelings of guilt usually have two components. The first of these is the "wrongdoing": you feel that you have either done something wrong, or haven't done something that you should have done. The second component is the "self-blame": you blame yourself for doing this wrong thing, and *feel* that you are "bad" because of it. That's the culprit! It is the concept of "badness" that creates the guilty feeling. If you feel bad about doing something wrong, this is normal and understandable. But when you start telling yourself that you *are* bad, guilt follows.

What if other people tell you that "it's okay?" This may not help. Your feeling of guilt may have nothing to do with what others tell you or what they think. Even if they disagree with you, these are still your feelings. Remember: Your guilt comes from the feeling that you are a bad person, rather than from feeling bad about what you have done. Is it fitting to label yourself as a bad person or blame yourself because you've done something wrong? Even if you have done something wrong, it's better to label that particular behavior as bad, rather than yourself.

Is the behavior that you are blaming yourself for really that terrible or wrong? Does it justify the feeling of badness that leads to guilt? In Nell's case, then, she felt guilty because of her MVP. Does that make sense? Did she make it happen? Of course not. Nell might feel better, therefore, if she emphasized the good times she still could have with her husband, rather than the specific activity that might not be as feasible.

WHAT IS VS. WHAT OUGHT TO BE

Guilty feelings about problems with spouses or children or the lack of time to spend with loved ones are very common for people with MVP. On the other hand, some people tend to feel more guilty about the inability to advance in their careers or to fulfill their job responsibilities the way they feel they should. How about Connie, age thirty-eight. She felt guilty because she was not able to work as hard at her job as she used to. She therefore earned less money, not enough to provide all of the luxuries she and her family would have enjoyed. Feeling under pressure, Connie tried to work harder to earn more money, which in turn made her feel worse physically. This created the guilty feelings. She felt less positive about herself, feeling she was letting her family down. How does one cope with these feelings?

Do you see a difference between the way you are doing something and the way you think you should be doing it? If so, you can really feel the old guilt horns! How do you work this out? Major union/management problems would seem to be easier to solve! Can you work harder or do more? If you can, then do it. If not, try examining your day-to-day goals for working and living. Check to see if these goals are practical, considering what you can and cannot do because of your MVP. Try to take more pride in what you can do. Although most people hate hearing that "things could be worse," this phrase is quite true. You might not be able to do anything at all. If you concentrate on the things you can do and place less emphasis on what you can't, your feelings of guilt will diminish. You'll feel a lot better.

Changing the emphasis in your thinking will also help you to lessen the gap between what is and what ought to be. This is what led to these guilty feelings in the first place.

Does this approach work only for working people? No. It applies to anyone who feels guilty because of falling short of expectations and desires. Jack, a seventeen-year-old student, was feeling guilty because he was unable to devote the amount of time to his schoolwork as he previously had, or as he would have liked. He was more and more reluctant to go to school because he was so frequently unprepared, and he missed a number of school days because of MVP. The guilt he felt affected his schoolwork even more.

How might Jack cope with these guilty feelings? It might be beneficial for Jack to speak to each of his teachers and explain how mitral valve prolapse was affecting him, cautioning his teachers that his physical condition might occasionally affect his schoolwork, and that his attendance might not be as good as it had been. At that point, it would be helpful to discuss possible methods for making up for this, such as extra projects that he might be able to work on when he was feeling up to it, or alternate arrangements for testing (to try to show his teachers that, even with less time available for studying, he was still interested in succeeding in class). By working with his teachers and setting more realistic goals, the feelings of guilt related to having MVP and its effect on his schoolwork should decrease.

TALK IT OVER

It is very important to discuss how you feel about your condition with others who may be affected by it. It is helpful to talk over feelings with the important people in your life, to share concerns, and to try to figure out solutions to problems. Noreen, age twenty-five, had enjoyed a very active social life before being diagnosed with MVP. In addition to going out on weekends, she and her husband would play racquetball with friends or participate in other social activities at least two or three evenings during the week. Now, because of the way MVP was affecting her, she had to restrict her activities. She just couldn't go out as frequently. She couldn't even play racquetball at all. Sometimes, she wouldn't want to go out even once during an entire week. Not only did she feel unhappy about her condition, but she felt extremely guilty at holding her husband back. She felt that he couldn't have a good time because of her. It would be helpful for

Noreen to discuss alternatives with her husband. Arriving at a solution, with her husband's cooperation, could effectively reduce guilt feelings and improve the marriage.

THOUGHTS CAN HURT, TOO

So far, we have been discussing how doing the wrong thing can lead to guilt. But it's not only "behavioral mistakes" that can lead to guilty feelings. Thoughts can also become upsetting enough to lead to guilt.

Sometimes, you may feel guilty without doing anything wrong. You may be merely thinking things that cause guilt. Suzie, a twenty-eight-year-old mother of two young children, was feeling terribly guilty. Why? Her thirty-year-old husband was spending many hours taking care of the kids and helping her with the housework. Suzie knew that her condition meant that she couldn't do what she used to, but she felt bad because her husband had to do so much. She was afraid that he would eventually start complaining. Should Suzie blame herself and feel guilty because of her condition?

In order to cope successfully with guilt, you must first focus on what led to the guilty feelings. Have you actually done something wrong? Have you really neglected something you shouldn't have? You may feel guilty about your thoughts or desires, rather than specific actions or behaviors. Recognize that, if you haven't done anything to lead to guilt, then you should identify those thoughts that are making you feel like a bad person. Change them. If you can learn to talk to yourself in a positive way, looking at your thoughts objectively and constructively, guilt can be reduced.

Frequently, as in Suzie's case, feeling guilty is related to seeing yourself as responsible for others' actions or behaviors. The more responsible you feel, the more guilt you may feel, especially if you cannot fulfill your responsibility. Frequently, just asking the question "why?" will point out that this thinking is unrealistic. That alone can help to reduce guilt. This is another reason why discussions with other important people are helpful. They may explain why taking the responsibility for someone else is inappropriate.

Be sure to place feelings of responsibility in proper perspective. There is a limit as to how responsible you should feel for others' actions or feelings. Nor are you responsible for having mitral valve prolapse, or for any restrictions this may place on you. Suzie should recognize that nobody was forcing her husband to take over household responsibilities. Suzie should not feel responsible for her husband's choice; being aware that she shouldn't can reduce guilt. Realize that when individuals are not forced into an activity, they participate out of choice and desire. The same holds true for this book. You are reading it out of choice and desire, aren't you?

"SHOULD" THOUGHTS

Among the most common causes of guilt are thoughts containing the word "should." "Should" is a dirty word! Examples of such thoughts are, "I should have been able to finish that job today . . ."; "We should have that party—all our friends have entertained us this year . . ."; "You should have let me do the dishes . . ."; "I shouldn't have MVP." These "should" thoughts imply that you must be just about perfect, and on top of everything.

When there is a difference between what you feel should occur and what actually does occur, guilt can result. You will become upset whenever you fall short of your "should." Should thoughts lead to guilt simply because they are not sensible, realistic, or justifiable? Should you blame yourself because the thoughts determine goals that you may not be able to fulfill?

Now that I've explained what you shouldn't do, what exactly should you do? In order to feel better and reduce feelings of guilt, it is helpful to reword your thoughts to eliminate "should" thoughts. Try to use less demanding words. Say, "It would be nice if I could finish that job today, but I can't," rather than, "I should finish that job today." If your physical condition is restricting your activities, you'll feel much more guilty when "should" thoughts remind you of unfulfilled obligations. If you have trouble changing the wording of your "should" thoughts, try asking yourself, "Why should I . . . ?" or "Who says I should . . . ?" or "Where is it written that I should . . . ?" This may help you decide whether you are setting up impossible requirements for yourself. It also can help you to reduce your feelings of guilt.

Let's say, for example, that you are thinking of having a party because all your friends have invited you to get-togethers. Ask yourself why you should? Is it because the "Party Rulebook" tells you that, if you don't have a party, your friendship license will be revoked? Is it because, if you don't have a party, your friends (some friends!) won't invite you to their homes anymore? As you think about the realistic answers to these questions, it will be easier to realize that you don't have to have a party. Although it would be nice, it is more acceptable to wait until you feel better.

THE CONSEQUENCES OF GUILT

So far, we've been discussing what leads to guilt, how you may feel, and how you can try to adjust your thoughts and behaviors to feel better. But what happens if you have not yet been successful in eliminating guilt? People who feel guilty frequently act in negative ways to hide from these feelings. There may be a tendency to indulge in "escape" behaviors, such as drinking or excessive sleeping, which do not deal with problems head-on but, instead, attempt to push them away.

The first step toward improvement is to look past the escape behavior and identify whatever is causing the guilt. Consider what can be done to rectify the problem causing the guilt. At the same time, try to eliminate any escape behavior, recognizing that it is only a cop-out. It is possible, however, for there to be no clear-cut solution to the events or feelings creating guilt. Don't give up because no complete solutions exist. Look for partial solutions. These may not be as desirable, but they can still help to reduce guilt by reminding you that you are trying to improve the situation.

OTHER SUGGESTIONS

We've talked a lot about how thoughts and behaviors can cause guilt. But what if you just feel guilty and can't remember what you were thinking or doing to make you feel that way? How can you start using all these great thought-changing ideas if you don't remember what thoughts you want to change? Good question! In order to identify those "target" thoughts or behaviors, you might want to keep a brief, written log of feelings or activities that may have caused your guilt. Once you have written these things down, you can then begin figuring out how to change them, improving your outlook, and reducing your guilt.

Mary, age thirty-nine, had been feeling increasingly guilty recently but didn't really know why. By keeping a log, she noticed that besides complaining of fatigue almost all the time, she had been arriving at work late on a regular basis. She wasn't aware of how frequently she had been late, and she had always been proud of her punctuality. The log helped her to see that she needed to improve her morning routine in order to be more punctual. As she worked on this problem, her guilt lessened.

What about those negative thoughts that lead to guilt? It can be very helpful to try to turn these thoughts around, making them more positive and guilt-free. For example, let's say that you feel guilty because you believe you are a bad parent. Ask yourself if you have ever done anything that a good parent might do. Just about every parent can come up with something. This starts the process of eliminating your "bad parent blues." The idea is to turn your mind's negative thoughts into reasonable, positive ones. This way, the feeling of guilt will not take a stranglehold!

A FINAL GUILTY THOUGHT

Guilt is a very destructive emotion. If you feel guilty, it can certainly interfere with your success in coping with MVP. By becoming aware of how guilt develops, you have a much better chance of effectively employing coping strategies to reduce guilt and its negative effects.

12

Stress

Stress. Stress! Every time you turn around you're reading or hearing about stress. The word "stress" is used very frequently these days. What exactly is stress? Stress is a response that occurs in your body. It helps you mobilize your strength to deal with different things happening in your life. It describes those things that create nervousness, anxiety, tension, anger, or an upset feeling. Actually, these are all parts of stress, rather than the same thing.

Many things occur each day that require you to adapt. These are the "stressors." All the changes that occur in your body when something (the stressor) provokes you are known as the "stress response."

By now, everyone knows that stress can play a role in causing or exacerbating virtually every medical problem. MVP is no exception. There are times when stress can trigger MVP symptoms. What kinds of stress are we talking about? There are many, including emotional stressors such as work-related problems, marital disputes, deaths in the family, and so on, or physiological stressors such as injuries, illnesses, or accidents.

IS STRESS GOOD OR BAD?

A certain amount of stress is normal and necessary. Stress helps you to "get your act together," and prepares you to handle your life in the best possible way. Now you're probably thinking, "So why do I always hear people talking about how stress can be harmful?" When people talk about the harmful effects of stress, they are referring to situations where there is too much stress. Then it can become destructive. If left unchecked, it can eat away at you and drain all your energy.

Reasonable amounts of stress can be handled. In fact, they can even be helpful. This chapter, however, is concerned with harmful stress, the kind that can hurt if not controlled.

Esther, a thirty-eight-year-old housewife, was under pressure. Her husband was bringing his boss home for dinner. She had just started feeling some chest pain, and because she knew she got exhausted easily, she nervously paced herself as she prepared the meal so she wouldn't get run down. The stress she felt was tolerable, that is, until the phone rang. Her husband called telling her that, due to an emergency business meeting that evening, they'd be arriving two hours early! Esther's stress was no longer tolerable!

With mitral valve prolapse, you may experience stress for many reasons. For example, pain alone can cause stress. Chest pain, especially, can cause stress. Your concern about how your condition may affect you can cause stress. Worries about not being able to fulfill responsibilities can be stressful. Problems with medication or dietary changes also may be stressors. Any one of these, or others, can provoke a stress response.

Regardless of how damaging excessive stress may be, stress is something that still cannot be totally eliminated from your life. It is around all the time. The difference, of course, is not whether or not stress can be eliminated, but how it can be most effectively dealt with. Therefore, the goal is to improve the way you deal with stress. You want to change the situations that cause you stress, and even more importantly, change the way you respond to it. You want to try to improve the way stress affects your body as well as your mind.

WHO FEELS STRESS?

Everyone experiences stress. Nobody escapes it. But since stress can be positive or negative, learning how to respond positively will lead to a more successful emotional and physical life. If you have a hard time responding to stress, this won't be easy. Some people are more vulnerable to negative stress responses than others. Are you?

YOUR UNIQUE STRESS RESPONSE

Every person has a unique way of responding to stress. Stress control or management (effectively managing the way you respond to stress) is within your reach. Your pattern of response depends on a number of things: your upbringing, your self-esteem, beliefs about yourself and the world, what you say to yourself, and how you guide yourself in your thoughts and actions. The degree to which you feel in control of your life plays a role in your stress response. The way you feel physically and emotionally, and the way you get along with people, are also a part of it. To sum it up, everyone's method of dealing with stress is unique and individual, and depends on a complex combination of thoughts and behaviors.

Stressor + Interpretation = Stress Response

The way that you respond to stress depends on the "chemistry" between two factors. The first factor is the stressor, or the outside pressures. What is going on around you that is creating the problem? The second factor is how you interpret the things that are going on around you. It is the interaction of the stressor and your own internal reaction that determines your response to stress. (Sound familiar? Yes, it's the same "formula" that can be applied to anger, depression, and all the other emotions.)

This equation has important implications for coping with stress. Why? You're realizing that it isn't just the environment that causes your stress response, but also the way you interpret the stressor. Some stressors in the environment would produce stress in anybody. What would happen, for example, if somebody pointed a knife at your throat? Calm acceptance, or a stress response? Get the point? It's important to learn how to reduce the number of stressors that negatively affect you, as well as improving your reaction to those you can't avoid.

Body Vs. Mind

How do you respond to stress? Like one's response to anger or other mobilizing emotions, there are two main ways: physically and cognitively.

What happens physically? If you experience a stressful situation, the circulatory system speeds up. Blood is pushed rapidly toward different parts of the body, particularly those parts necessary to protect you. Because the blood supply is diverted toward these essential parts, the supply to the digestive system is usually reduced. As a result, the digestive process slows down, making it work less efficiently.

You may tremble or perspire. Your face may flush. You may feel a surge of adrenaline flowing through your body. Your mouth may become dry or you may feel nauseous. Your breathing may become more rapid and shallow. Your heart may begin to pound. Your muscles may become tight, creating headaches, cramps, or other painful reactions. Sounds lovely, doesn't it?

A cognitive response includes the way you think and feel. Your cognitive or emotional response to stress may not be as visible. You may start worrying, getting upset, fearing the next "event," and so on. You may not be able to concentrate as well. Your attention span may be reduced. You may have trouble learning something new. You may be afraid to do things. You may withdraw or feel nervous. You may lose confidence in yourself.

You may become more aware of any unpleasant physical responses, and this may make you feel even more stressed. For example, if you feel stress and respond with shallow, rapid breathing or heart palpitations, being aware of these physical responses may create even more stress. This can lead to feelings of panic. Most people respond to stress in both ways, although it is possible for you to respond in only one way.

What's Your Response?

Each person is vulnerable to stress in his or her own unique way. For example, certain parts of your body may tend to be more vulnerable and, when stressors occur, it is these parts that feel the effect. For example, have you ever felt extreme intestinal discomfort and automatically clutched your stomach because of stress? Or have you ever endured a painful headache? Or have you experienced a time (or times) that stress has played a role in your mitral valve prolapse, or in another medical illness or condition that you've experienced?

Chronic or prolonged stress puts a severe strain on your body. When your body is strong, it can fight off most foreign invaders, bacteria, and germs. As a result, many diseases can be avoided. But prolonged stress puts such a strain on the body that your defense mechanisms may break down. This, in turn, makes your body more vulnerable to the very problems you'd like to avoid!

Have you heard of the "fight or flight" syndrome? Animals do this when they feel threatened. The animal prepares to either fight or run away, a purely physical response. You will not see an animal standing there, scratching his head, and thinking about what should be done! But humans have the unique ability to think and reason! Lucky us! So this also becomes something we must work on to improve. (By the way, researchers feel that this is one of the main reasons why human beings are susceptible to so much stress-related physical illness. By thinking, instead of acting, we may not be dealing with stress as effectively as we might.)

When does stress lead to physical problems? When you can't respond to stress in a way that eliminates it, the stress continues unabated. Being unable to do anything about it may cause even more stress, creating a vicious cycle. This can take its toll on your body.

THREE RESPONSES TO STRESS

When a stressful stimulus occurs, you will most likely respond in one of three ways. You might respond immediately and impulsively without giving enough thought to a better response. You might not respond at all, and either try to ride it out, or become so frozen that you are unable to respond. Or, you may respond to stressors in a well-planned, organized, and effective manner. If so, you may not even need this chapter! But if not, read on!

HOW TO DEAL WITH STRESS

Stress may affect the circulatory system in many ways. Because of this, stress management is a very important part of any MVP treatment program. Remember: Stress can affect a person both psychologically and physiologically. Stress can be managed and controlled, but it cannot be eliminated. Stress will always exist. You can deal with the amount of stress you endure and with its intensity, but you'll never be able to make it go away. Stress management techniques can help you to better deal with both types of stress responses.

For a person with mitral valve prolapse, it is especially important that stress be controlled. Why? Although stress by itself does not cause MVP, it certainly may play a role in exacerbating mitral valve prolapse symptoms.

So what can you do? Let's begin by mentioning the wrong ways of responding to stress. These are the ways that don't help you: smoking, getting drunk, using drugs, overeating, and overactivity. Not only will these activities distract you or delay the effects of stress, but they also can hurt you.

So what should you do? Try to learn new, more appropriate ways of dealing with stress than the methods you've been using. Relaxation exercises and regular exercise can be very helpful as part of stress management programs. It is also important to learn to work on your thinking regarding stressful situations. By thinking more appropriately, reducing upset feelings, and improving your perspective, you can help to reduce stress. One of the most important goals of stress management is to improve your feelings of being in control, feeling responsible for your actions and thoughts.

Relaxation Procedures

The best way to start controlling stress is by using relaxation procedures. Try the "quick release" method discussed in the introductory chapter of this section. Other successful methods of relaxation include meditation, self-hypnosis, imagery, or even a warm shower! Deep breathing alone can help to eliminate tension from the body, slow down the heart, and create a sense of well-being.

Learning to relax can be helpful in reducing the amount of stress you are experiencing. It will give your body a chance to rest and recuperate as well. A stronger body can deal more effectively with the ravages of stress (or of life)! Relaxation also will help you to sleep better. Have you been experiencing any sleep problems since the onset of your condition?

Pinpointing Stressors

Stress is a type of energy that needs release. It can be handled either positively or negatively. In order to learn how to cope successfully, you must first identify your stressors. What, specifically, is causing you to feel stress? Maybe you're having a hard time with the symptoms of mitral valve prolapse. Maybe you're concerned about the reactions of others. Or maybe you're tired of worrying about your heart. These are all possible MVP-related stressors and, of course, there are plenty more.

What if you're not sure what's causing your stress? How can you figure out what it is? One way is to keep a record of your activities and experiences. You might want to use a numerical ratings scale, such as one called the SUD Scale. SUD stands for Subjective Units of Disturbance. How does it work? Ratings on this scale range from 0 to 100, depending on the amount of stress you're experiencing. Use 100 to represent the most extreme and disturbing stress, and 0 to represent no stress (total and complete relaxation). Then rate your activities, experiences, and thoughts on the SUD scale. The ones with the higher SUD numbers are the ones causing you the most stress. For example, loud, blasting music from your teenager's radio might be rated a whopping 85!

Identify Your Stress Reactions

Once you have begun identifying your stressors, you must then become completely aware of your responses to them. Are they more physiological or psychological? What parts of your body seem to be the most vulnerable? What kind of reactions does your body show? Does your attention span suffer? Do you get heart palpitations? Do you start losing confidence, or feel like you're slipping? As you become more aware of this, you will develop a more complete picture of your unique stress response. You'll be able to recognize the stressors that affect you and how you react to them. You'll then be better able to decide whether or not you should modify your behavior in responding to the stressor.

What's the next step? Once you recognize which stressors are negative, try to determine whether or not you can eliminate them. If you can, start figuring out how to do it. Removing the source of stress is an obvious and logical way to manage stress. Develop a plan of attack. This might include a number of alternative strategies, all designed to remove or minimize the impact of the stressor. Taking a sledge hammer to that radio might be great, if you could lift the hammer!

But what happens if you can't eliminate the source of your stress? You'll then have to work on your means of interpreting what's going on. You'll have to work on your thinking and your responses in order to manage stress. In such cases, changing the stressor is out of your control, but changing the way you react isn't. You might want to use some of the suggestions discussed in the chapters "Depression" and "Anger." The use of systematic desensitization, discussed in the chapter "Fears and Anxieties," also can be beneficial. Many techniques for changing your thinking have already been discussed in previous chapters.

Physical Stress Relievers

Certain physical activities can be great for stress control. For example, some people can relieve tension or stress by driving. As long as the driver continues to observe safety rules, driving can be very relaxing.

Exercise

Another important way of dealing with stress is by exercising. As you'll read later, exercise is not only important in helping you deal with stress, it can be a very healthy component of your treatment program for mitral valve prolapse. Regardless of how MVP is affecting you, there are still exercises you can do to help yourself control stress. Virtually any type of exercise can be effective. Anything that allows for a release of tension is ideal.

Keeping Busy the Fun Way

Hobbies or other leisure activities can be very helpful. They can divert your attention away from the stressful situation, directing it toward something more enjoyable. These activities also will help you feel productive. A lack of productivity may be one of the stressors giving you problems in the first place!

Another technique for dealing with stress is sleep. Some people have difficulty sleeping when experiencing high levels of stress. But if possible, cat naps, short naps, or even prolonged periods of sleep may be possible and can help reduce stress.

IN CONCLUSION

What are your goals? If stress is interfering with your achievement of these goals, then your stress response is negative. Learning how to control stress is a very necessary part of successfully achieving your goals, as well as successfully coping with mitral valve prolapse.

13

Other Emotions

The emotions we've covered so far in this section are not the only ones, of course. Worry, for example, is a basic emotion. What might you worry about? Have you got a month to discuss all the possibilities? You've probably worried about the future, what your life will be like, how life will change because of mitral valve prolapse, among countless other things. What other emotions enter into the picture? This chapter will discuss four other emotions common in life with MVP: boredom, envy, loneliness, and upset.

BOREDOM

Hopefully, by this time, you are not so bored that you have stopped reading! As long as you aren't bored, let's talk a little about boredom! What an empty feeling! It's one of the worst feelings anyone can experience. It has been said that more problems and serious tragedies come from being bored than from any other single condition.

Why are you bored? There may be no meaningful activity going on, no stimulation or excitement. Your life may seem to be going nowhere. Nothing is challenging you, and there's no incentive to do anything. Because you weren't born bored, you must have learned to be bored. You weren't always bored, and even now you are not always bored. There are still certain things that hold your attention from time to time. Right?

Is MVP Boring?

I bet you never thought of MVP as boring. But it can be, primarily because of any restrictions your condition may impose on you. Many activities that provided enjoyment for you in the past may seem to be out of reach. You may not even want to bother starting something new, telling yourself that future activities may be restricted because of mitral valve prolapse.

Celia was too tired to leave her house. She couldn't go shopping, she couldn't meet friends for lunch, and she was fed up with the garbage on television. Was Celia bored? You bet she was! Her friend suggested that Celia go along with her to take a course in interior decorating, since Celia had a lot of talent in this field. But despite her enthusiasm, she decided not to because she didn't want to start something she felt she couldn't finish.

So what should you do? Don't let your condition cause you to give up on life. Distinguish between what you can do and what you can't. If you do have to curtail any activities because of MVP, you'll do so. If you have to drop an activity, you'll drop it. But you don't have to eliminate all activities from your life simply because you feel you won't complete them.

"Unboring" Yourself

What can you do about it? The first step is to analyze why you are bored. What is causing the boredom? Obviously, figuring this out will help you to determine how you can improve things. Then you'll want to see what you can do to add some interest to your life. But don't feel that you must push yourself to enjoy something. Forcing yourself to become amused rarely works. You may find that activities you used to enjoy have become artificial and uninteresting. You may no longer get any pleasure from them. That doesn't mean, however, that you should give up, and not try to do anything. You do want to try some new activities that will make your life more interesting. Don't limit yourself to those things that used to interest you. Preferences change. Try things that never interested you before, because maybe now they will spark an interest in you.

Learn Something New!

One of the most effective weapons against boredom is learning. The mind is like a sponge, always ready and willing to soak up more information and knowledge. Select a potentially interesting topic you don't know much about. Try to learn something about it. You may want to begin by simply going to the library and reading some books on the topic. Maybe you'd like to enroll in an adult education course. Often, boredom quickly disappears once you are involved in something new. Learning is a great way to do this.

You can also become bored if your social life is not the greatest. What can you do about this? Once again, try to learn something, especially by taking courses of some kind. Aside from the mental stimulation you'll get from such learning activities, you also may meet interesting and challenging people. Increasing your circle of friends is a good way to fight boredom.

Anticipation!

One of the best ways to fight boredom is to always give yourself something to look forward to. It doesn't matter how small this may be. It can be as simple as reading a chapter of a good book, writing a letter, making that phone call you've been looking forward to, watching a television program you've been excited about, or meeting somebody special for lunch. Try to schedule something to look forward to every day. This way, even if part of your day seems boring, whether you're doing menial chores or just resting to build up your strength, you will at least have something enjoyable to look forward to. You won't give the weeds of boredom a chance to take root!

Goal-Setting

Set goals for yourself, both short-term and long-term. Boredom can arise from plodding along with no purpose in life. Having something specific and tangible to shoot for can be helpful in fighting boredom. This doesn't mean you'll never be bored. You may still have to give yourself an occasional kick in the derriere to keep moving toward those goals. But isn't it better to have something to shoot for than to have nothing at all?

ENVY

You've heard the cliché, "The grass is always greener. . . ." If you have MVP, you're probably envious of others who do not. This is understandable. You may be envious of other people who are able to do more than you can.

Envy can be a destructive emotion, because it's a type of self-torture. It can be very painful. You're constantly putting yourself down and comparing yourself with the better qualities of somebody else. You feel inferior. This can lead to other feelings as well, such as anger or depression.

Why is envy a problem? Because it shows that you are not satisfied with being yourself. You want to be like somebody else. You want to have what somebody else has. Does this mean that the other person has a happy life? Is that person happier than you in every way? You may have MVP, but this doesn't mean that everything else about the other person's life is superior. Stop and think for a moment. I'm sure you can come up with some areas in which your life is better!

Is Envy a Positive Emotion?

In general, emotions usually serve a purpose. Emotions such as anger and anxiety mobilize you to prepare to handle their sources. On the other hand, envy is a destructive emotion. It does not have the positive qualities that other emotions may have. But maybe you can find something positive in envy. If you recognize that you're envious, analyze the reason why. Try to change this by concentrating on yourself and your own attributes. Don't let envy get you down.

How Does Envy Occur?

Basically, there are four conditions necessary for you to feel envy. First, you feel deprived. You feel like you can't have something that you want or need. This doesn't just mean money, pleasure, properly working valves, or even health! Envy is an intense feeling that involves more than this. It seems like your feeling of need lies deep inside. Second, somebody else has whatever it is that you feel you're missing. Third, you feel powerless to do anything about it. You feel totally unable to change the circumstances that have made you envious in the first place. This helplessness causes you to feel more and more bitter. This makes you even more envious! Fourth, there is a change in the relationship between you and whatever it is that you envy, be it person, object, or situation. You no longer simply compare yourself with the other, but feel fiercely competitive. You may begin to feel that the only reason you don't have what you would like is because somebody else does.

If you feel envious, is it necessarily the same kind of envy that everyone feels? No. There are actually two types of envy. One is an envy of tangible things (cars, boats, homes, friends, and so on). The other is less tangible, such as pleasure or health. If you have MVP, you may still have many tangible things. You may still have a family, a car, and a place to live. You may still have a job. But the fact that you're not happy with your medical condition makes you envious in an emotional sense.

What Can You Do?

Concentrate on being yourself. Increase the positive benefits and enjoyments you can get out of life. Why worry about comparing yourself with somebody else? What's that going to do? Sure, your mitral valve may not be functioning the way you'd like it to. But that doesn't mean you can't enjoy life as much as somebody else can. Set up reasonable goals for yourself, considering other things you have and how you feel. Then you can say that you're living your life as enjoyably as anybody else. This is more possible when you do not compare yourself with somebody else. Remember, you are you. Concentrate on making the best of your own life.

LONELINESS

There is a difference between being alone and being lonely. Being alone simply means that there is no one else with you. This can be either good or bad. But being lonely is usually a downer. If you feel lonely, it doesn't really matter whether or not there's anyone with you. What's more important is where you stand with other people. Loneliness is a sad, empty feeling, but one that is usually created by you.

Why might you feel lonely? You may feel left out if you can't spend time with others the way you used to, either because you're not feeling well or you can't do what others want to do. Maybe you feel lonely because you feel other people don't understand your condition. You may simply feel different from others. You may decide to change some of your relationships because you have a hard time dealing with these people. Does that mean you're happy about these changes? No.

It's hard to be lonely. Not just because you feel bad, though. It actually takes effort to make yourself lonely—it doesn't just happen. And you have to work hard to keep yourself feeling lonely. There are many opportunities to be with people. As a result, loneliness usually occurs out of choice rather than accident. In order to be really lonely, you'd purposely have to exclude everyone around you from your life. You'd always have to be on your guard, protecting yourself from the horrible possibility of making a new friend!

Why Be Lonely?

Why might you want to be lonely? There are four reasons. First, if you're lonely, you probably enjoy being lonely. This may contradict what you complain about to everyone else. If you're lonely, it's because you like it enough to not do anything about it. Second, if you're lonely, it's because you're hard to please. You may feel that you don't want to even bother trying to create new relationships because no one meets all of your requirements. Third, if you're lonely it may be because you feel you must be lonely. You've resigned yourself to it. You tell yourself that this is part of the price you have to pay for having mitral valve prolapse! Fourth, and probably most important, if you're lonely it may be because you're scared. You're afraid to develop new relationships. You're afraid to make yourself vulnerable because you're afraid of being rejected. You may recall previous experiences that did not work out the way you wanted. You don't want to relive the hurt and pain.

Break Your Lonely Ways

Reading about this isn't easy, especially if you are a lonely person. Why? It's not easy to think that maybe you did this to yourself! But there is still a light at the end of the tunnel! Recognize where your feelings of loneliness come from. Admit to yourself that maybe it's not such a great feeling and you should try to change it. There are things that you can do.

Don't Be a Pusher

The first step is to stop pushing people away. Unseen vibrations are given off, telling people that you don't want them around. These intangible vibrations reduce your number of acquaintances, adding to your feeling of loneliness. This must stop. You have to learn to give off positive vibrations, the kind that welcome people instead of chasing them away.

Contact!

Once you start giving off new, more positive vibes, you'll want to make more friends. How can you meet people? You can start by getting involved in some kind of organization. This type of activity usually attracts people who are interested in being with others who share a common goal. Because you have MVP, you may want to become involved in your local chapter of the American Heart Association. There you may meet other people with similar concerns (helping you to better cope with medical problems). In addition, you may be able to find ways of helping others. This is a great way to develop friendships.

Try getting involved in a new learning activity or hobby. Take adult education courses, for example. This will help alleviate loneliness as well as boredom. Invite people to your home, but pace yourself so that you don't become exhausted. Most importantly, be receptive to the people that you meet. Try to see the good in everyone. Don't reject someone simply because there are some things that you don't like.

If you work at conquering loneliness, you'll feel much better about yourself and about your life. It will make life more enjoyable, even though you have MVP. Give yourself and others a chance, and your feelings of loneliness will disappear, regardless of the limitations your condition has placed on you.

UPSET

Are there times when you feel unhappy but you're not really depressed? You might feel uncomfortable but not anxious. You may not know exactly what's bothering you, or what to do about it. On the other hand, you may know exactly what's wrong, but you just don't like it. You can do things, but you'd like things to feel differently. You may feel mixed up, confused, disturbed, agitated, or shaken up. This is typical of feeling upset. Can you get upset because of MVP? Be serious, now!

When things happen to upset you, you may try to push them out of your mind so that you can adjust as slowly and as comfortably as possible. But eventually, you'll certainly want to come to grips with it.

Feeling upset is similar to experiencing other "motivating" emotions. They propel you to do something. So what should you do, now that you're all motivated? Try to figure out why you're upset. You do want to do something about it. There's probably something in your life that is out of sorts. Things are not moving along smoothly. Something has upset the "apple cart."

Rose was upset. A thirty-four-year-old mother of four, she had just completed her latest car-pool adventure and was about to relax in front of her favorite soap opera on the tube. She had a gnawing feeling that things just weren't right, and this upset her. She knew she was upset when she found that she couldn't enjoy her program. My goodness, she had been hooked on this show for almost twenty years! But she decided to turn off the T.V. and figure out what was upsetting her. After at least four commercials-worth of thought, she realized that it was her soap opera that was bothering her! She felt that the characters on the program, despite all of their script problems, were better off than she was. They didn't have MVP, she did! None of them needed medication, only she did! As she thought about it, however, she realized that perhaps she was making something out of nothing. Actors and actresses have their own problems. So what if she also had something she must learn to live with. She had proven to herself that she could live and be happy, even with MVP. She quickly noticed that she was feeling much better. In fact, she was able to turn on the television and breathlessly catch the last few minutes of her show!

Once you explore your upset feeling, you can act on this in much the same way as you do in attempting to resolve other emotional concerns. If you can identify the source of your upset, then plan a strategy. Otherwise, recognize that you can't, and move on.

PART III
Changes in
General Lifestyle

14

Coping With Changes in General Lifestyle— An Introduction

So you have to make changes in some aspects of your lifestyle because of mitral valve prolapse? Yes, that is all part of the "package." How may MVP affect you the most? You may not be too happy if it forces you to change your lifestyle dramatically and you're not able to cope with it!

But changes may occur in anyone's life for a number of reasons. If you got a new job, you might have to wake up at a different time, go to work in a new direction by a new form of transportation, or "survive" on a higher salary. If your new job required you to move, you would have to meet a whole new group of people. If you got a new car, you'd have to get used to its new gadgets, as well as new quirks. If there was a new addition to the family, you'd have to get used to crying, changing diapers, and night feedings.

In your case, mitral valve prolapse is a new addition to your life! Although it may be hard for you to try to lead a normal life when you know your condition may never be totally cured, you're not (or shouldn't be) aiming for perfection. You just want to feel better, enjoy life, and do what you can. That's reasonable and achievable.

Because you have MVP, it's important that you work through concerns that you have about modifications in lifestyle. If your lifestyle has to change in order to deal with MVP and live most comfortably, then any changes that have to take place have to be worked through and accepted. There are always things that you can do to improve the way you live and deal with this condition.

Because mitral valve prolapse can affect work, family life, sexuality, social activities with friends, finances, and other aspects of day-to-day living, it's important for you to learn how to cope with changes in lifestyle. Even though, in many cases, these changes may be minimal, you might as well understand what you can do to cope with any changes that do occur.

Your lifestyle is of your own choosing. You'll automatically take many different factors into consideration when determining what your lifestyle is and what you want it to be. You can decide how full you want your days to be. You may also decide to put things off until you "feel better." But in the case of mitral valve prolapse, why wait? Why not try to see what you can do right now to improve the quality of your life, even while you're learning to live with mitral valve prolapse?

SELF-CARE

It's very important to learn how to identify and interpret the symptoms you are experiencing and what they mean. This is important in learning to take care of yourself. For example, if you have chest pain or palpitations, what should you do about them? When should you seek proper medical advice, what are the appropriate times to check out these symptoms, and what actions should you take if there is an emergency? You want to know how to modify your lifestyle, how to take medications correctly, when necessary, and how to follow your doctor's prescription.

MAKING SOME CHANGES

A good way to change your lifestyle is to look for ways that you can make things easier for yourself. This may allow you to continue doing much of what you want to do, without putting as much pressure on your body. In fact, as you make changes (at your own pace), you'll feel even better because you'll probably experience less discomfort. You'll make changes in lifestyle that can help you to reduce or avoid discomfort, as well as save your energy.

For example, try to spread out your most taxing activities. Why is it necessary to do all the house cleaning in one day? Spread it out. Pace yourself. Make sure you include rest periods during the course of the day so you can "recharge your batteries."

GETTING USED TO THE CHANGES

What are some of the factors that will determine how well you'll adapt to changes in your lifestyle? There are many. For example, what were you doing before you were diagnosed with mitral valve prolapse? How satisfied were you with your major vocational (job) and avocational (leisure or recreation) activities? How much education did you have? How supportive were the people close to you— both family and friends? How has your condition affected you, both physically and emotionally? These and other questions play a role in determining how you'll adjust to MVP, its treatment, and any changes it necessitates. But that doesn't mean your hands are tied. You can improve the way you deal with virtually any factor.

Your head may be spinning, fearing changes that may have to take place in your activity schedule, job, or social relationships. You may also be apprehensive about dealing with physical discomfort, body changes, and medication. In fact, you may even be concerned that you won't be able to perform your normal chores and responsibilities. This concern is not unusual. Most people with mitral valve prolapse do feel this way. But feelings improve. Being aware that you can do more also helps.

How About Denial?

What happens if you decide not to comply with necessary changes in lifestyle? This may indicate that you're trying to "deny" your problem. Denial is a very common coping strategy. Believe it or not, there are times that denial can be a positive technique. How? It can be helpful by keeping you from dwelling on problems that aren't helped by dwelling! In other words, if there's nothing you can do to make a situation better, why keep thinking about it?

But denial has its negative side, too. What if denial keeps you from doing what you need to do? For example, what if you don't get enough rest, or you don't eat properly, or you don't take all your medication, or, or, or . . . ! This is destructive denial, and it can hurt you. Hopefully, the fact that you're reading this book in the first place shows that you're not really denying inappropriately. But continue to stay on top of this.

Yes, there may be some changes in your lifestyle. But why assume that all of them have to be negative? Isn't it possible that some of them might be for the better? Maybe you were such a hard worker that you never spent enough time with your family. If you have to cut back on your work schedule because of mitral valve prolapse, perhaps you'll enjoy the increased time you'll have to spend with your family. It's possible that some of the medication you may use to control mitral valve prolapse will help to also control other pesty problems that have been troubling you for awhile (whether related to mitral valve prolapse or not). Learning to take better care of yourself will pay off in the long run. So don't convince yourself that your life is ruined because you have mitral valve prolapse. Always look at the positive in any situation. We'll be discussing how to deal with as many of the negatives as possible.

GUIDELINES FOR CHANGE

Here are some general guidelines for living with mitral valve prolapse that make sense if you need to modify your lifestyle:

- Be aware of how your body feels. How is it reacting to things you are doing? Act accordingly.

- Build on the talents and activities you can still enjoy (and there'll be plenty of them).

- Pamper yourself a little. Learn that you don't have to do everything for yourself. Accept help from others when necessary, and don't "overpush" yourself to do anything.

- Be more protective of yourself. Follow normal routines you have established to get the proper amount of sleep, exercise, and nutrition. Try to avoid contagious diseases, injuries, and infections.

- Remember: you are the most important ingredient in the recipe for successful adjustment to having MVP. Help yourself.

Coping with changes in lifestyle forms a very important part of the process we call rehabilitation. What is your goal? To help yourself to live as normal a life as possible despite your condition.

The remainder of this book will address many of your concerns about lifestyle changes. The remaining chapters of Part III will be concerned primarily with changes in the things you do, the way your body feels, and the way mitral valve prolapse affects you. So read on, and let's get your act together!

15

Physical Symptoms

Any chronic medical condition can affect you in two ways—physically and psychologically. We've discussed how to cope with your emotions, now let's focus on the physical effects of MVP. They do play a major role in your psychological adjustment to having MVP.

There are a number of possible physical symptoms with MVP. You can't do something about all of them, but some of them can be treated, and also can be helped by changing things about yourself or your life. Even then, some symptoms may just go on. With those, you must learn to simply accept them. You must learn to live with them, even if you don't like them. That may seem like a tall order, but what choice do you have? After all, you're still the same person inside. So why not concentrate on things you *can* do something about. Deal with physical symptoms as they come, when they come. Don't anticipate the worst since the worst rarely happens.

HOW DO THESE SYMPTOMS PRESENT THEMSELVES?

The MVP symptoms that most often get you to go to the doctor include palpitations, chest pain, shortness of breath, anxiety, and fatigue. In so many cases, these symptoms just seem to appear out of the blue, with no apparent explanation. Sometimes, though, something may seem to have provoked them.

When you notice these symptoms, you may feel very frightened. A feeling of impending doom is not uncommon (after all, the heart is involved!)! Anxiety or panic attacks may be common. If so, coping skills or psychotherapy may be helpful, as well as the use of medication, if necessary. Many times, just hearing the doctor tell you that what you're feeling is very common and will not result in a cardiac catastrophe will be sufficient to help you to calm down and feel better. Any other treatment that is necessary will focus on the physical symptoms that are being experienced.

Let's discuss four of the more common and anxiety-provoking symptoms of MVP: fatigue, chest pain, palpitations, and shortness of breath. If there's anything you can do about them, suggestions will be offered. If not, at least you're learning more about the symptoms, and you're becoming aware that you're not alone in experiencing them.

FATIGUE

Do you become more tired, more easily? Does your bed seem to be your favorite place in the whole world? If so, you're not alone. Fatigue (yawn!) is one of the most common and unpleasant problems for individuals with MVP. Your body simply may not be able to do what you want it to do. Fatigue encompasses the loss of that "get up and go" feeling, not only tiredness or sleepiness. You feel so tired that you just can't complete the things that you want to complete.

There are two possible times when you may feel tired. In some cases you'll feel tired following some activity or expenditure of energy. But the other, more puzzling time, comes by surprise. You may not have done anything tiring when all of a sudden your body decides to go on a rest cure! You feel like the energy has drained right out of your body, like water from a leaky radiator. It seems almost impossible for you to do anything at all.

How do you feel when fatigue hits? You may feel like a rag doll, with arms and legs that are so floppy and limp that you just can't move them. You may feel like a marionette supported by strings, after the strings are cut. You may feel like a balloon that has popped and just collapses in a whoosh. Or you may quiver and tremble uncontrollably, like a bowl of Jell-O (flavor does not matter). Whatever it feels like to you, fatigue is hard to deal with.

But that's not all. On top of your frustration comes the disbelief of people around you. That's right—because fatigue is not "observable," they may just not believe you when you complain of being tired. They may not be able to understand how you could go from being active and on the ball to being tired and listless in such a short period of time.

One of the most upsetting things about fatigue is that you never know when it's going to hit you. You may be going along just fine, and then bang! All of a sudden it feels like somebody has just pulled the plug! You may awaken in the morning feeling fine, and then have fatigue hit quickly during the day. On the other hand, you may awaken in the morning feeling very tired and find that your energy builds up during the day.

The fatigue of mitral valve prolapse may or may not have anything to do with the stress you're under or the amount of activity you're participating in. The degree of fatigue you experience can vary widely. Without doing anything different, you may fluctuate from feeling strong enough to do virtually anything to feeling too weak to do anything at all.

What Causes Fatigue?

Why does fatigue occur? It is not completely understood. One theory relates to the functioning of the autonomic nervous system. It is suggested that because of the imbalance in the autonomic nervous system that often accompanies MVP, the blood vessels do not dilate or constrict properly. This can alter the proper blood flow to the entire body. If the blood flow feeding and nourishing the large muscles of the body is restricted there may be a build-up of a chemical called lactic acid. This lactic acid accumulates because the large muscles are not getting sufficient oxygen or nourishment. Fatigue is one of the results of a higher-than-normal production of lactic acid. There are other theories too, such as the fact that cardiac arrhythmias, anemia, or even the use of betablockers as a medication to control symptoms, may cause fatigue.

The cause of fatigue may not be totally physiological. Fatigue can be caused by doing too much! Or it can occur even if you haven't been too active. Too much activity, or even too much rest may be a cause of fatigue. Fatigue also can be due to other emotional factors. Psychological variables such as excessive stress, anxiety, or depression also may contribute to fatigue.

One of the problems if you are experiencing chronic fatigue is that you may feel less able to be active. This inactivity results in even more fatigue. Unless something happens to break this chain, you may become more and more poorly conditioned.

Fatigue also may result if you participate in less exercise because of fears of exacerbating your condition. You may be concerned about physical exertion. You may fear that any exercise will be dangerous (it needn't be, if you build up your strength and stamina gradually and properly). Because of these apprehensions, however, you may quickly become out of shape. You may feel more comfortable doing less. And, of course, the less you do, the more out of shape you become! In addition, doing less increases the cycle of doing even less. Fatigue breeds lack of activity.

Most people think of fatigue as negative. This is not always the case. It can be positive. How? Fatigue is your body's way of telling you that you need rest. If you didn't feel tired, you would push yourself too much! Then you'd certainly feel the effects. So if you feel fatigue, you should listen to your body.

Trying Anti-Tiring Tactics

What's the best way to cope with fatigue? Rest. (Clever!) Allow yourself longer periods of time for sleep at night. In addition, try to arrange for at least one or two brief rest periods during the day, preferably in the late morning and late afternoon. This may help replenish some of your energy.

In addition, the best strategy for dealing with fatigue depends on the nature, as well as the cause, of the fatigue. It depends on how much fatigue you are feeling and how it's affecting your body. But regardless, you'll want to make sure you get the proper amounts of rest to nourish your body.

Although rest may not make fatigue problems disappear, it certainly can help. If fatigue is a message saying that your body is unable to do as much as you want it to do, rest is certainly an important way to gain more control. One problem, however, is that too much rest can lead to more fatigue! This can start a vicious cycle. So you'll also want to make sure that you're getting enough of proper types of exercise. Proper exercise helps to break the cycle of fatigue and out-of-shape deconditioning.

Fatigue also can be reduced by efficient planning and pacing. Figure out exactly what your responsibilities are. Schedule activities so that you're not doing too many strenuous things in a row. Make sure you intersperse rest periods with any strenuous activities you need to do. And be flexible. You can never be sure when you're going to have energy, or when you're going to feel too fatigued to do anything.

Learn how to pace yourself during your normal routines. You may have to change your general lifestyle in order to maximize your energy level. Know your priorities. Focus on the top priorities while you still have the energy. In this way, if fatigue sets in, it will be the less significant activities that need to be delayed.

Things you used to do that took extended periods of time may have to be shortened or eliminated. For example, were you a professional shopper, one who normally spent six hours in the shopping center? This may not be possible (or appropriate!) now.

What about the times that you know that your fatigue is emotional? Try to determine what emotional reactions are contributing to the fatigue. For example, fatigue could be due to depression, boredom, worry, or just unhappiness. Then you can work on improving these feelings.

CHEST PAIN

Chest pain can be a very uncomfortable problem with MVP. Although chest pain is a very common symptom, it is still not completely understood exactly why it occurs. Some people think that pain may be caused because there is a lot of tension on the muscles of the valve. The release of certain hormones also may increase stress and create more discomfort. Some theorize that this chest pain is caused by a spasming in the muscles of the heart. The spasming may coincide with the clicking of the leaking mitral valve. However these are just theories.

In addition to it being very common, it also may be very frightening. One of the most frightening feelings anyone can experience is a tightening, gnawing pain in the chest. "Uh, oh," you may panic, "heart attack!" Research reassuringly states that the pain experienced as a result of MVP is *not* the same as the chest pain experienced by individuals who may be having a heart attack. The pain that one experiences when having a heart attack results from muscle tissue dying because the heart muscle is not getting the appropriate amount of oxygen. However, this may not be much of a comfort to you if you're still frightened by MVP chest pain!

How about the comparison between MVP chest pain and that of angina pectoris? The critical manifestations of these pains are different. Chest pain in MVP usually occurs on the left side, usually is brief, and doesn't necessarily have anything to do with effort-laden activity. All these characteristics are different from those of angina attacks.

Although the chest pain of MVP is not the same as heart attack pain or angina pain, it is real pain. Because it may occasionally be severe, it certainly can be very frightening. It's important to remember that, although the chest pain is real, it doesn't pose an imminent threat to life. On the other hand, any pain that is experienced as a result of MVP is pain that should be brought to the attention of your doctor. One of the doctor's most important responsibilities is to monitor these chest pains, and to help you deal with any pain that does occur.

What Can You Do?

No treatment, not even medication, has helped every person with chest pain. But that doesn't mean that there is nothing you can do about this pain. Because chest pain is such a common symptom of MVP, and because there are (fortunately) so many things you can to reduce pain, you'll read more about a number of these techniques in the chapter on, appropriately, Pain!

HEART PALPITATIONS

Palpitations are another common symptom of MVP. With individuals with mild MVP, the symptoms most often experienced, if any, are occasional palpitations.

In general, palpitations, along with chest pain, are the symptoms that most often get people to go to the doctor! They may create anxious feelings that a heart attack is imminent. Actually, palpitations are usually due to an arrhythmia, or an erratic heartbeat, in the ventricle. The palpitation sensation in the chest may feel like a butterfly-type fluttering. People sometimes describe it either as feeling like skipped beats or rapid heartbeat. In general, palpitations are not serious, and they don't require treatment, but they certainly can be anxiety-provoking! So you'll want to learn how to cope with them.

People with MVP are often very much in tune with their own heartbeat. They may feel that they notice it all the time. They are often surprised to find out that people without MVP are not aware what their heartbeat feels like, never notice it, and really are not concerned.

What Can You Do?

As with chest pain, bring your symptoms to the attention of your doctor. Together, you can then decide which treatment is appropriate. On some occasions, medication may be considered, but in many other cases, non-pharmacological techniques like relaxation and working on your thinking may be sufficient.

SHORTNESS OF BREATH

Shortness of breath is another common symptom of MVP. However, it is not understood exactly why it occurs. (Sound familiar?) Shortness of breath may have an impact on you because of the limit it imposes on your activities. Obviously, if you experience shortness of breath, it's going to slow you down and keep you from doing as much as you want. In addition, experiencing shortness of breath can certainly be anxiety-provoking! As a result, you may decide to decrease your activity level. This anxiety can in turn trigger additional shortness of breath! This can become a very unpleasant vicious cycle.

What Can You Do?

Learning smooth, rhythmic, breathing along with slow exhalations can be helpful. Breathing should be done in slower, more deeply formed, breaths. Shortness of breath can be helped by techniques designed to improve muscle control during breathing. Using abdominal muscles, for example, can help you to increase confidence in your breathing.

Relaxation and imagery also can be helpful in dealing with breathing problems. Reducing muscle tension can smooth out breathing problems. And peaceful, relaxing imagery, where you know that you're breathing efficiently, can help to slow down breathing, deepening it as well. Any of these techniques are also important because they can help you to feel more in control. A feeling of control helps to reduce the anxiety that can lead to more problems.

Smoking and Shortness of Breath

No discussion of shortness of breath, or helping you deal with the symptoms of MVP, would be complete without mentioning smoking. It's amazing how many people there are, with all different types of chronic medical conditions, who still smoke. Despite all the research that smoking is hazardous to one's health, that it can cause new medical problems, and that it can exacerbate existing medical problems, many people with MVP continue to smoke. Smoking is one of the lifestyle factors that must be controlled in order to improve your physical condition with MVP. If you smoke, and you've fully decided that the time has come to stop, there are many resources to pursue. Speak to your physician, your pharmacist, or to organizations like the American Heart Association or the American Cancer Society. Go to the library—there are many books that can help you. (You don't have to buy the books; by the time the book is due, you should already have stopped!)

A PHYSICAL FINALE

This chapter has discussed some of the more common physical symptoms of MVP. Although not pleasant to think about, you do want to learn how to cope with MVP, right?

Any combination of symptoms, chest pain, palpitations, and shortness of breath, for example, may frighten you to the point where you'd probably be less active. You might feel that this is one way to insure that nothing terrible is going to happen. You may still decide to decrease your activity, despite reassurances from your doctor that you are not having a heart attack. But the problem is that this would result in a decrease in the tone and physical strength of your body. And it may even increase the likelihood that more of these negative symptoms are going to be experienced!

This is a destructive cycle. So you can understand why one of the most important goals of treatment is to break this cycle. This will help you to start slowly to improve dealing with any MVP symptoms you're experiencing. You'll also build the confidence that you can continue to lead a strong productive life.

16

Pain

Ouch! (Just getting you ready for this chapter!) Might you experience pain with mitral valve prolapse? Yes. Unfortunately, this can be a common symptom of MVP.

What can you do about your pain? How can you cope with it? The best way to cope with pain is to get rid of it! That makes sense! To see if you can do this, it's first necessary to identify the cause of the pain. Once this is done, treatment can be aimed at eliminating the cause. But there's a problem. In some cases, it may be impossible to do anything about the underlying source of the pain. So pain itself, rather than the cause of the pain, is the most important concern. What does treatment aim to accomplish then? Relief from pain!

GETTING STARTED

How do you start? First, be aware of your pain. Sure, you say, when I experience chest pain, I'm not aware of anything *else!* But being aware of your pain is important so you'll learn to recognize whether the pain is something you can (and should) handle yourself, or if it's serious enough to be brought to your doctor's attention. Remember: If in doubt, check it out. Inform your doctor about the pain. Together you can work out the best ways of dealing with it.

It is important for you to recognize that MVP-related pain is real. All too often people may say that the pain is in your head and that you're imagining it. That's because *they* are not experiencing it! Still, this can be very damaging to self-confidence. Fortunately, though, the pain that occurs as a result of MVP is not the same as angina, or pain that might indicate potentially dangerous heart problems.

WHEN DOES PAIN OCCUR?

Many factors may contribute to your pain. You'll want to try to control any or all of these factors in order to manage it. Remember that pain can be exacerbated by both psychological and environmental factors. Although pain may initially be physical, emotions can quickly worsen the pain. So pain may result from stress, fatigue, or depression.

Stress causes you to tense your muscles. It may make it more difficult for you to relax. This can increase the degree of pain that you're experiencing. If you're fatigued, you may feel more pain because your tissues aren't getting the rest they need to repair themselves. Depression may cause you to feel more pain because it's on your mind more than it would normally be.

When you're in pain, this may increase the degree to which you experience stress, fatigue, or depression. This can lead to more pain, creating a vicious cycle.

It is also important for you to identify any other factors that may exacerbate the pain. Other factors such as anxiety or boredom can cause pain to be perceived as more pronounced. Because of this, it makes sense to try to do what is possible to reduce these problems.

TREATMENT FOR PAIN

There are four traditional categories of treatment for pain control: medical (using medication), surgical, physical (physical therapy), and psychological. In general, all four therapies work by interrupting the transmission of pain messages before the brain receives and interprets them. In MVP, surgery to replace the valve may be done in some cases, although this is a very rare occurrence. But when surgery is performed, it's not done merely for pain relief! So let's discuss the other three categories and how they can help you relieve your pain.

MEDICAL TREATMENT

Medical treatment for pain generally involves medication. In many cases, this can effectively decrease or eliminate the pain. But sometimes discomfort will continue, despite the use of medication. More information about the different medications used in treating mitral valve prolapse will be discussed in the next chapter.

Although medications can be helpful for pain, it is probably better if you are not dependent on them. Pain medication works by blocking pain signals. This may be dangerous if there are things going on in your body that the brain is not becoming aware of because of pain-blocking medication. For example, pain medication may interfere with the brain's receiving messages indicating cardiac overload and fatigue. Another problem when pain killers are used for a long period of time is the chance that there may be damage to your kidneys.

Unfortunately, one of the facts of life with mitral valve prolapse is that not all pain may be able to be eliminated. So it may be necessary for you to learn other techniques for dealing with pain.

NON-MEDICAL TECHNIQUES

Some physical therapy techniques can be useful in dealing with MVP pain. Learning a proper balance of rest or exercise can be very helpful. Taking warm baths or placing warm moist packs on the chest may improve feelings of relaxation, comfort, and well-being.

A goal of treatment for MVP is to reduce the heart's workload. Exercise can help, even though it may seem like it will actually increase heart activity. But as the heart muscle becomes stronger, it will more efficiently be able to pump blood throughout the body. And a more efficient heart doesn't work as hard! Less load, less pain! The chapter on exercise will discuss in detail how it can help your life with MVP, as well as provide suggestions for how to implement an exercise program.

Other than physical therapy techniques, some people look to psychological techniques such as imagery, biofeedback, yoga, hypnosis, and relaxation, or even acupuncture or chiropractic, as pain control sources. Last, but certainly not least, it's very important to maintain a positive attitude.

PAIN CONTROL RESOURCES

You can learn how to employ techniques for controlling pain from physicians, physical therapists, mental health professionals (such as psychologists who may specialize in certain pain control techniques), or other health professionals. Or you may want to read some of the many books on pain that can be found in bookstores and libraries. Many techniques for pain control can be applied at home, although in some cases they may work better if you learn them in clinics or centers.

Despite the effectiveness of many pain control techniques available today, it's important to consult your physician to make sure that any or all of the techniques you're considering are appropriate for you. Consider your condition in making sure that any techniques you're thinking of using are not dangerous for you.

ALLEVIATING THE PAIN PSYCHOLOGICALLY

There are many nonmedical factors that may influence the experience of chest pain, including anxiety, depression, and fatigue. Because of this, these factors need to be controlled as much as possible. But isn't pain purely physiological? Rarely. It's usually a combination of physiological and psychological factors. Although you may be experiencing true physiological chest pain, your mind is very much involved in determining exactly how much it hurts.

What does all this mean? If medication or other medical intervention doesn't help alleviate your pain, you can still relieve some (if not all) of it by working on your mind's awareness of it. Read on to find out how this can be done.

Relaxation Techniques

One of the goals of pain relief techniques (as well as MVP treatment programs in general) is to reduce the workload of the heart. Relaxation techniques, for example, can decrease muscle tension and improve circulation. Relaxation decreases the body's need for oxygen. All these things help to decrease the heart's workload. Relaxation can help you to reduce your overall levels of pain, as well as to deal more effectively with pain.

Relaxation is the opposite of tension, and tension can actually increase your pain. There are a number of different types of relaxation procedures including progressive relaxation, meditation, autogenic training, hypnosis, and deep breathing procedures.

Let's discuss other psychological techniques to help control pain, such as imagery, biofeedback, and changing your way of thinking.

Imagery

There is a relationship between your mind and the way you feel physically. Much research has proven this. Scientists have also found that bodily functions previously thought to be totally beyond conscious control (autonomic is the scientific term—we've talked about the autonomic nervous system, remember?) can be modified using psychological techniques!

One popular technique is imagery, or the process of conjuring up pictures or scenes in your mind. In practice, imagery has been beneficial in helping to deal with a host of physiological and psychological problems, including headaches, hypertension, depression, and pain. In many cases, imagery procedures have worked well in combination with prescribed medication for treating medical conditions.

Here's how imagery works. Sit in a comfortable chair or in bed and get into a relaxed position. Lights should be dimmed, and outside sounds or noises minimized. Try to avoid interruptions. Breathe smoothly and rhythmically, allowing your body to release tension and relax. Then imagine a scene of your own choosing, trying to make the image as vivid and real as possible. This scene can be used therapeutically to help you feel better.

Wendy was experiencing a sharp pain in her chest. She was instructed to relax and then develop an image of what this pain looked like. She imagined it as a very sharp knife being jabbed into her chest. Others may feel like their chest is being hit by a hammer, or that they're having dozens of pins stuck into them. Whatever imagery you develop, it should be as vivid and detailed as possible. Wendy was then instructed to reverse what was happening in the image: She imagined the knife slowly being removed from her chest, and a soothing, healing cream being applied. Finally, the knife was completely out. She was then able to relax and her discomfort was eliminated.

There are other images you could use to reduce chest pain. For example, you could imagine cool air being blown inside your chest, or a soothing lotion being gently massaged on the affected area, or a warm bath melting away the pain. These images can be used anywhere. (Have you ever taken a bath on a bus?!) With regular use, they can help you feel better. Imagery is really restricted only by your creativity. A good book on the subject is *In The Mind's Eye* by Arnold Lazarus. See if your public library or local bookstore has it.

Imagery is a key component in hypnosis. Hypnosis may be helpful since it can be quite effective in the area of pain control. Many good books on clinical hypnosis are also available in libraries and bookstores.

Biofeedback

Biofeedback combines the procedures of relaxation and imagery with the use of measuring instruments, usually electronic ones. These machines let you know what's going on physiologically (giving you feedback) in your body (bio). The devices, which are connected to different parts of your body, provide moment-by-moment information about any changes that are taking place.

Biofeedback can help you learn to control certain automatic body functions by obtaining feedback from certain measurement techniques. You can learn how to voluntarily control internal functions of your body that you may have previously thought were involuntary or uncontrollable. Blood flow or activities of the brain are among your body's automatic functions.

One of the main advantages of biofeedback is that there are usually signals that you can hear or see. Electrodes are either taped to your skin or attached in some other way. They pick up responses that are transmitted to the biofeedback unit as electrical impulses. These impulses are then translated into sounds or lights that you can observe. In this way, you may receive continuous information about body functions such as blood pressure, heart rate, muscle tension, or skin temperature. Using this information, you can develop different types of imagery so that you can learn how to control your internal responses.

Gayle was experiencing a lot of pain, so her physician suggested she try biofeedback. A machine measuring muscle tension was attached to where she was experiencing the pain (in much the same way that electrodes from an EKG machine are connected. There is no pain, and you won't get jolted!). As she attempted to relax the area, the machine gave her instant feedback as to whether she was really relaxing, and to what degree. As she became aware of her lowering tension, she learned what mental images were helping her to relax. She could then continue using these images on her own, without the machine, to help her relax and control some of the pain.

What kinds of biofeedback equipment may be used? Most frequently, machines can be used to measure skin temperature, pulse, blood pressure, the electrical activity resulting from muscular tension, or electrical activity coming from the brain.

Not only may biofeedback be helpful in reducing MVP-related pain or discomfort, but it also may be helpful in stabilizing some of the imbalance of the autonomic nervous system. Further research is still necessary.

Coping Psychologically

There are other factors that can contribute to the intensity (even the very existence) of your pain, including your emotional state, the attention you pay to the pain, and the way the rest of your body feels. Obviously, as you pinpoint which of these factors does play a role, you can begin improving the way you cope with pain.

Where do you start? You'll want to do everything you can to decrease fear, stress, tension, and other negative emotional factors. All of these may make you more aware of your painful physical state. Anything you can do to relieve anxiety and tension (including psychotherapy, if necessary) should help you to cope better with any pain.

How do you reduce the amount of attention focused on your pain? Of course, the more time you have to think about it, the worse it will seem. So try to divert your attention. Develop other interests that require concentration. You can always come up with thoughts or activities that will distract you from painful thoughts. One very helpful "activity" might be to get involved with a support group for people living with pain. Examples of such organizations are the National Chronic Pain Outreach or the American Chronic Pain Association. They have many chapters throughout the country, and more are always forming. It can be great to know that you're not alone in trying to cope with pain. Who knows? You may even get some great ideas that will help to reduce the pain you have to live with!

AN UNAGONIZING CONCLUSION

Unfortunately, it may be that you will have some pain because of mitral valve prolapse. But don't throw in the heating pad! Realize that the pain need not last forever. A lot can be done, both medically and psychologically, to help deal with it.

17

Weight Changes and Diet

Food, glorious food! Or is it, "Food, who needs it, food!" Are you eating less now, and enjoying it less? Or are you eating more and, possibly, gaining weight as a result?

Research has shown that MVP symptoms can be somewhat greater if you are overweight. Therefore, it makes sense that any person who has MVP and who could benefit from losing some weight, should. Even individuals who are more slender could benefit from a diet that is high in energy. Everybody needs fuel to energize the body. Individuals with MVP are no exception.

If you do have a weight problem, don't put all of the blame on mitral valve prolapse or your medication! Your weight may increase or decrease, or your appetite may change, and this fluctuation may have nothing to do with MVP. (It's easy to blame anything that is happening on mitral valve prolapse. Some people, physicians included, may do that.) Maybe your weight is fluctuating because of binges over the weekend! Maybe you've gone to some food orgies! Maybe you're retaining water, or maybe emotional crises have caused you to overeat. One of the most important things you can do to help stay as healthy as possible is to eat properly and keep your weight at an appropriate level.

Any weight control program designed to help you with MVP, or with life in general, is usually not successful if it just focuses on dieting alone. The best way to lose weight is to modify your diet to some reasonable (rather than drastic) degree and to increase your activity level. And emphasize good nutrition! For individuals with

MVP, good nutrition is the first important step in an effective comprehensive program to help you successfully live with the condition.

WHAT ABOUT DIETS?

Is there any particular diet that is most appropriate for mitral valve prolapse? There is no specific diet just for people with MVP. If your doctor feels it would be helpful for you, it may be suggested that you try a reducing diet, a salt-free diet, a low-protein diet, or a combination of the three. Other types of diets may be suggested as well, depending on your overall medical health.

A proper diet insures that you consume all of the necessary vitamins, minerals, and supplements. Regardless of any specific diet plan recommended for you, nutrition is very important in controlling symptoms of MVP. So there are some very important dietary considerations to keep in mind.

What are the most important dietary recommendations for individuals with MVP? Eliminate caffeine, eliminate or minimize sugar, limit your intake of fats, and increase your intake of fluids.

Caffeine

Why is caffeine a problem? Caffeine is a stimulant. Caffeine is found most often in tea, coffee, and some carbonated beverages. It is also found in chocolate and certain over-the-counter medications.

Remember that the autonomic nervous system is extremely sensitive to all drugs. Caffeine is no exception. Caffeine often gives a sudden boost to the autonomic nervous system. The reason for this is that adrenaline is released as a result of caffeine's stimulation. Then after this boost, there is a drastic drop off. A roller-coaster effect is created. This is not good for the autonomic nervous system and, as a result, not good for anybody with MVP. If you remember that balance, or a level state of equilibrium, is very important if you have MVP, you'll understand why the disequilibrium caused by caffeine should be avoided.

If you have been using caffeine excessively for a long period of time, don't try to stop it all at once. Try gradually substituting caffeine-free beverages or products. Caffeine, like any other drug, can be addicting. You're better off tapering off slowly. And as with any other drug, if you feel that caffeine is a problem and you need to taper off, discuss it with your doctor. Make sure that any major changes you think should be made are done only under a doctor's supervision.

Sugar

Sugar, like caffeine, can have a devastating effect on the autonomic nervous system. Like caffeine, sugar can also cause a physiological roller-coaster effect. If you eat something containing sugar, this stimulates the body into producing increased levels of insulin and adrenaline to compensate. When insulin and adrenaline circulate in the bloodstream, the blood sugar level drops significantly. It often drops lower than it was before you ate the food containing sugar in the first place!

A low sugar level is what creates feelings of hunger. When you get strong hunger feelings, it won't be long until you're going to eat again! And since so many foods that we eat contain sugar, a roller-coaster effect results.

Complex carbohydrates are much more important than simple sugars and starches in your diet. Why? The amount of energy used to burn and properly utilize food determines how much of the food is wasted and how much of the food is useful. The more energy it takes to use the food, the better the food is. Simple sugars require very little energy to digest. It is relatively simple for simple sugars to be broken down and burned. On the other hand, complex carbohydrates require much more energy and time to digest and break down. This helps the body to better utilize these nutrients.

Don't be surprised if you have difficulty reducing the amount of sugar in your diet. Sugar is also addictive. Many people have had difficulties decreasing the amount of sugar in their diets. Your goal, remember, is not to necessarily eliminate all sugar from your diet. Rather, you want to reduce the amount that you take in, as well as how often you consume sugar.

Fats

It is also important to reduce your intake of fats if you have MVP. Virtually everyone, whether they have MVP or not, can benefit from a reduced fat intake. Most of the fats that people consume are loaded with "baddies" that increase the risk of heart disease and other types of medical problems.

One of the "baddies" is cholesterol. Cholesterol creates the material that clogs arteries, leading to many different types of heart disease. Although the amount of cholesterol you need or that can be harmful is still in question, most studies recognize that cholesterol is something that must be properly controlled.

Understanding cholesterol involves knowing the three types of substances that make up cholesterol. They are called lipoproteins. There are three categories of lipoproteins: high density lipoproteins (HDL), low density lipoproteins (LDL), and very low density lipoproteins (VLDL). High density lipoproteins seem to be the healthiest type for you to have. But the most important statistic seems to be the ratio of these three types of lipoproteins in your body. Often your doctor will want to find out what your lipoprotein level is by requesting a test called a lipid profile. Once the levels are measured, the ratio will be determined.

Certain types of fats, the "saturated fats," increase the amount of cholesterol in your body and should be avoided. Saturated fats include all meat and dairy products, such as whole milk, butter, cheese, and eggs. The oils highest in saturated fat are the tropical oils— coconut, palm, and palm kernel. Another highly saturated fat source is cocoa butter, the oil used to make chocolate.

Other types of fats can lower cholesterol. "Monounsaturated fats," found in most foods but mainly in vegetable and nut oils (such as olive, peanut, and canola), will lower cholesterol. "Polyunsaturated fats," found mainly in nuts, oils from plants, seeds, and soybeans, also will lower cholesterol, but if consumed in excess also may lower the protective lipoproteins, HDL's. Keeping an eye on what you consume and how it will affect your cholesterol is a good idea for sound nutrition. Speak to your physician if you have any questions.

Fluids

Many individuals with MVP have problems with body fluids. If your mitral valve is not functioning properly, the blood may not be pumping throughout the body with proper pressure. There can be a decrease in circulating blood volume because of this low blood pressure. This can lead to fatigue and a decreased sense of well being.

One way to counteract this problem is through exercise. This improves both your conditioning and your circulating blood volume. The other way to counteract this problem is by consuming lots of fluids. Fluids help to maintain good blood volume, and also improve energy levels. The best fluids to consume are water, decaffeinated beverages, sugar-free sodas, and fruit juices.

HOW TO GET STARTED

To begin modifying your diet to help energize your body (and lose weight, if necessary!) to deal with MVP, keep a food diary. Write down everything you eat, so you can then analyze the quality of food you are taking in. The first modifications you'll want to make will focus on increasing the energy foods, especially the complex carbohydrates. You want to decrease fatty foods, which can make you more sluggish, and the foods that have empty calories. Try to identify which foods you eat that have too much sugar, salt, caffeine, or fats. You'll want to change these foods for foods that are more energizing, nutritious, lower in calories, and better for you.

Most nutritionists these days recommend that the most healthful diets should be made up of approximately 50 percent complex carbohydrates, 20 percent proteins, and 30 percent fats. Specific details on the best foods to consume are really beyond the scope of this book. But any library or bookstore has excellent resources on nutritional diets to help best energize your body.

A FEW EXTRA TIPS

What else can you do to lose weight and maintain proper nutritional balance if you have MVP? Make sure you eat a well-balanced, variety-packed diet. Having meals made up of tasty complex carbohydrates, proteins, and fats will help to best give you the energy you need as well as to keep you feeling satisfied until the next meal.

Eat regularly. Try to regulate the process of keeping food in your stomach. If digestion occurs regularly, without long periods of time between big meals, it keeps the blood sugars from fluctuating wildly, as they might if you were to go long periods of time without food and then short periods during which you were overloaded with food.

Include physical activity with any weight modification program in order to increase your metabolism and tone your body.

Limit alcoholic intake. Remember that individuals with MVP are highly sensitive to drugs. Alcohol is a drug and can affect the person with MVP even more adversely than it would affect someone without MVP. In addition, alcohol has empty calories, and can stimulate the heart.

LET THE EATER BEWARE!

Because diet is on everybody's mind these days, it has become a favorite subject of quacks. You may hear of miracle remedies involving certain types of dietary modifications that are "destined" to cure your physical symptoms. Be very careful of such claims. Check out their nutritional merit, and be sure to consult your physician.

The moral? Eat healthy, eat in moderation, and enjoy!

18

Exercise (And Rest)

Two important components in your effort to live more comfortably with mitral valve prolapse are rest and exercise.

REST

Rest is important if you have MVP. It helps you to avoid wearing yourself down. It also helps you to maintain an alert, active state.

It is very important for anybody who has MVP to learn to recognize an appropriate balance between rest and activity. Some people are clearly able to understand and identify this balance very quickly. Others have to learn the cues that they receive, both from their body and their environment, in order to determine the best possible balance between rest and activity.

Occasional rest periods may help you to feel strong for the remainder of your day. However, if you feel very tired too often, this may be your body's way of telling you that you need additional rest periods. So pay attention!

Yes, rest is important. But too much rest can be as dangerous as too little rest. You may feel even more tired. The more rest you get, the more you may want, and this causes a vicious cycle.

There are differing opinions regarding how long you should rest. Your physician, along with the old reliable trial-and-error, will help you to determine how long you should rest. You'll consider how uncomfortable you are, your lifestyle, and other aspects of day-to-day living.

EXERCISE

Many people with MVP do not do well with exercise. This may be because they're not in the best shape. Or maybe they're afraid to exercise because of possible chest pain. And, of course, there's that commonly held aversion to the discipline of exercise! But exercise may be a helpful component in your life with mitral valve prolapse. Why? What are the benefits of regular exercise? There are a number of them. Exercise can be helpful in keeping your body trim. You'll want to keep your muscles firm, firm, firm, which is better than flab, flab, flab!

Exercise also can help your body systems to work efficiently. A person who participates in regular exercise has more energy, is better able to handle stress, usually has fewer physical complaints, experiences less anxiety and depression, sleeps better, experiences the aging process slowing down, concentrates better, has fewer aches and pains, and so on. Exercise can build and maintain muscle tone, reduce pain, improve the efficiency of your cardiovascular system, help you to sleep better, improve your digestion, help you to control your weight, reduce fatigue, and increase energy levels. Don't you wish it did all this instantly?

There are so many good things that can come from exercising, how come not everybody does it? For many people, exercise ranges from extremely boring and avoidable, to moderately unpleasant. Only a small percentage of people really and truly enjoy regular exercise. (Is that you?) So, the best goal is to try to focus on exercises (and exercising environments) that can be as close to pleasant as possible! This will enable you to keep more easily with your commitment to regular exercise.

You'll need patience. Most exercise programs really do not show results for three or four weeks. Individuals with MVP may notice that progress takes even longer because of their condition. But patience is important: You will see the results, as long as you stick to it. Of course, if you give up too early. . . .

Those who attempt to accelerate an exercise program to bring about faster results will end up suffering more than they will benefit. The first few weeks of any exercise program may be the most difficult. This is because you are trying to integrate new habits with your routine. There may be many times when it is easier just to not exercise than to push yourself to do so. However, it's better to commit yourself and make this a part of your normal routine. The habits will continue to keep it as part of the routine, and the benefits will be wonderful.

Problems With Exercise

Many people with MVP do not physically do well with exercise. If exercise tests are given to them as part of their medical treatment, for example, they do not do well on these tests. Although this is fairly common, not everyone experiences this.

In many cases, poor results on exercise tests do not have anything to do with the individual's desire. It may be that physiological fatigue sets in more quickly in these individuals. On other hand it may be because the fear of additional heart problems builds up. Because fear is so commonplace in those with MVP, less and less is done. This is what leads to the deconditioning process.

Deconditioning is a phenomenon that results from being less and less active. Your muscles grow weaker and, over time, you have less and less energy. What are the symptoms of deconditioning? The symptoms of deconditioning are very similar to those of MVP itself, including shortness of breath, rapid heartbeat, and increased fatigue.

However, both fear and deconditioning can gradually be reduced. How? Through exercise! By embarking on a gradually building exercise program, you can slowly build up tolerance levels, increasing your capacity and ability to participate in these activities.

Exercise and Your Cardiovascular System

What exactly do we mean by cardiovascular fitness? In general, the main purpose of the heart and lungs is to circulate blood containing oxygen to all the cells and tissues in the body. This circulating blood also removes metabolic waste products from the cells. The muscles, so important in our normal functioning, are also nourished by this oxygenated blood circulation. Cardiovascular fitness, a smooth, effective operation in the circulatory system, enables all the cells and muscles of the body to use this oxygen more efficiently. As a result, there is less of a demand for effort on the heart and the lung. The heart is required to do less work.

Some people believe that the main reason for exercise is to improve the muscle tone of the heart, enabling the heart to beat more strongly. That is only part of the picture. (And certainly, in individuals who have experienced heart damage because of coronary artery disease or heart attacks, exercise is not necessarily going to improve the function of an already permanently damaged heart.) However, exercise does improve the muscles' ability to function more efficiently. This increase in efficiency decreases the demand on the heart, enabling the entire system to work more smoothly.

Everybody can benefit from more exercise, regardless of limits imposed by a medical condition. There are always more things you can do. But remember the need for a proper balance between rest and exercise. Only by trial-and-error can you really determine whether you are exercising or resting in the proper amounts.

Is Exercise Good Only for Your Body?

Exercise is as important for psychological well-being as it is for your body. Exercise gives you the feeling of being able to do something. It can build up your self-confidence. Have you lost some good feelings about yourself due to your medical condition? Exercise can help. It will restore some confidence in your body. Seeing improvement in your performance as a result of exercise also can build up your self-esteem. Exercise clears your mind, keeps you alert, and helps to control some of the unpleasant emotional reactions that may occur from time to time. Exercise can help to control stress, as well as emotions such as depression, anger, fear, and frustration.

Exercise can help you to sleep better so you'll feel better the next day. And unless you exercise alone, you'll enjoy some healthy social interactions—always good for the mind (as well as the body)!

Getting Started

Before any exercise program is begun, you should consult with your physician. Once you have decided to exercise, make sure you commit yourself to it. There is no benefit to be gained by exercising for a day or two, and then giving up. To benefit most from an exercise program, you'll want to do it regularly.

If your medical condition (or your anxiety) has kept you from being active, be prepared for something frustrating. When you first begin to exercise again, wow, will you be out of shape! That's not a put-down. Your muscles will need time to start regaining their strength. So any kind of exercise should be implemented gradually. The longer it's been since you've done any exercising, the slower your return should be.

Many individuals with MVP experience increased discomfort when they first begin their exercise program. Yes, you can expect to experience more fatigue and possibly a slight increase in discomfort when you first start exercising. However, at minimal levels this is to be expected, and really cannot be avoided. Discuss this with your doctor, so you'll feel reassured. You should not experience extreme discomfort when you exercise. If you do, stop immediately and consult with your physician. The slight increase in fatigue, and any aches and pains that you will notice, will disappear as you consistently participate in your proper exercise program.

Most individuals who start on an exercise program usually work together with their physician or a physical therapist to determine an exercise prescription. This is a good way to make sure that the exercise you do is healthy. And, it will help you to keep track of what you're doing and how it is helping you, so that you will continue to be committed to it. It cannot be emphasized strongly enough: Make sure that you have your medical professional's approval for any exercise program that you plan to follow.

Make sure that when you exercise, you do it properly, following proper guidelines and safety rules. Do not build up your pace too quickly. Let your stamina and your muscle tone develop gradually and it will stay with you that much longer. You'll want to follow a concept in exercise known as "the progression principle." This principle states that exercise should be started slowly, and as time goes by, the degree and intensity of exercise increases.

One of the most important concepts in exercise is "the overload principle." What this principle states is that you must put more effort into an exercise than you would normally do (the overload) in order to become more fit. Usually, the overload principle should be applied at least three or four times a week, for a minimum of twenty minutes, in order to really gain the benefits that you want in reconditioning the body. However, for some, exercising only three or four times a week is not even considered to be enough. They feel it's usually important to get some regular exercise at least five to six times a week. Be very careful about how you apply this principle. Consult with your physician. Remember, in MVP, heart overload is not something you want to do.

Exercising Caution

Not every exercise is appropriate (or even safe) for every person. So make sure you have your doctor's approval before doing any exercises. You may even want to undergo professional exercise testing, to see what you can and cannot do, and develop a program to build your abilities. Once you've set goals for yourself, you can start building up your exercise ability gradually. Don't exceed the moderation that's required.

You'll want to learn the difference between muscle soreness (which may be a normal response to exercise) and acute pain (which is a result of a particular exercise, and may either mean that you're overdoing it, or that you're participating in an exercise that's a no-no). The old adage, "No pain, no gain," is not really true if you have mitral valve prolapse. What you really want to do is enough exercise so that your muscles feel good each day. You're trying to improve both tone and strength.

If you get involved with a health spa or an exercise salon or anything of the sort, make sure that the professionals are well aware of your condition. But even so, make sure you consult with your physician about any prescriptions you may be given for exercise. Because as much as they say they know about MVP, they still may not know enough. You don't want to jeopardize your health.

Categories of Exercise

What are you trying to accomplish through exercise? That usually determines how to categorize it. In other words, exercise can be divided into aerobic exercises, range-of-motion exercises, muscle strengthening exercises, and stretching exercises.

Most exercise routines incorporate three components. The warm-up, where you start stretching to get yourself limber; the main part of the exercise routine, where you do your aerobic exercises, calisthenics, or anything of the sort; and then the cool-down period at the end.

Aerobic Exercises

Aerobic exercise is exercise that improves the way you utilize oxygen. These exercises require increased amounts of oxygen for prolonged periods of time. As a result of doing aerobic exercises for at least twenty minutes a few times each week, the way your body uses oxygen can improve. For example, your lungs will be better able to inhale and exhale, blood volume will increase, and tissues and muscles throughout your body will be better able to use the oxygen that is brought to them by the blood. Aerobic exercise does not necessarily require that you work harder when you are exercising. Rather, you'll just work longer.

Although, in general, people say that aerobic exercises should be maintained for at least twenty minutes, when you are beginning a program, you still do not want to overdo. So you may want to start with a sustained five- or ten-minute effort, and then gradually build that up as you have more confidence.

The key to aerobic exercises is that they be done for sustained periods of time, usually at least a few times a week. Good examples of aerobic exercises include walking, riding a stationary bicycle, climbing stairs, walking on a treadmill, aerobic dancing, swimming, and slow jogging.

Aerobic exercises can also be used to build up endurance. That's because these exercises are less beneficial for specific muscles but more helpful for overall fitness. They are usually a good complement to stretching, range of motion, and strengthening exercises, if these are appropriate for you.

Range-of-Motion Exercises

A joint's normal movements (in different directions) fall into the category "range of motion." Range-of-motion exercises stretch joints in various directions by manipulating the muscles attached to them. These exercises are not specifically beneficial for MVP treatment (although it can always be good to have limber joints).

Strengthening Exercises

Strengthening exercises, such as isometric or resistive exercises, increase the size of the muscle, but they do very little to help the cardiovascular system. In fact, the sudden change in energy exertion and blood pressure when strengthening exercises are used may not be a good idea for people with MVP, especially if their blood pressure is already unstable.

Stretching Exercises

Stretching exercises are done to relieve any stiffness or tightness in the muscles or tendons surrounding a joint. If joints are not being efficiently used due to inactivity, the muscles controlling these joints are not doing anything. This disuse will adversely affect the muscle, causing such problems as spasms, cramps, or decreased flexibility. Stretching exercises can help that problem. They're a good way to begin any exercise program.

Guidelines for Exercise Benefits

To be sure you derive the greatest benefits from an exercise program, there are certain guidelines that should be followed:

- Make sure you check with your physician before undertaking *any* exercise program. This way, you'll learn what's best for you, and medical supervision can be reassuring.

- Any exercise program usually should begin with a short warm-up period. Warm-up periods usually involve just stretching and limbering up and preparing the body for the more strenuous activities that will follow.

- You should try to participate in activities that emphasize good muscle tone rather than muscle bulk buildup. For example, walking and swimming are better exercises than weight lifting! It's also a good idea to have a regular exercise program, rather than exercising whenever "the spirit moves you"!

- Don't feel that you have to wait until any MVP symptoms go away before starting an exercise program. Starting sooner may even help you to feel better more quickly. But get professional advice and supervision.

- Develop your ability to tolerate exercises slowly. Because one goal of exercise programs is to improve your functioning, keep trying to increase the amount of exercise you do, but do this gradually. Too rapid an increase, or too intense an exercise program, may only increase the pain that you're experiencing. It also may decrease the benefits you derive from exercise, not to say that it won't decrease your *desire* to exercise!

- Anticipate minor discomfort from exercising. Remember, you're doing things that your body may not be used to doing! Some people feel it's a good idea to push yourself just a little (very little) beyond the level at which pain first occurs. This may help to increase your tolerance. But be very careful. Discuss it with your doctor. You may be told that if you experience too much discomfort or pain, or if it lasts too long, you should cut back. It probably indicates that you're overdoing! So listen to your body!

- Don't compare your exercise program to somebody else's. You wouldn't compare your doses or types of medication to somebody else's, would you (or should you)?

- If you decide to join a gym for your exercise program, be on guard against instructors who tell you they know "just what will make you feel better." They may know very little, if anything, about mitral valve prolapse. Better to come in with suggestions for exercise from your physician, and simply ask the instructor to see that you're following your program correctly.

- Commit yourself to your exercise program for at least two months. By this time, most people will see the benefits of what they've been doing, and will continue. This decreases the chance of being an "exercise dropout."

A Final Calisthenic

Exercise can either be extremely valuable or extremely harmful (or anywhere in-between!) depending on the care you use in approaching this activity. Because every person with MVP is different, there is no one set of exercises that is recommended for everybody. But everybody can benefit from something! Don't just jump in feet first. Use your head (not to jump in!). Speak to your physician or a physical therapist, start slowly, build up stamina, and enjoy as you feel better.

19

Medication

Changes in lifestyle, improving your mental attitude, modifying diet, and increasing exercise are all good ways of dealing with MVP. But these techniques may not always be enough. Another common treatment approach for mitral valve prolapse is the use of medication.

How do you know if your condition needs (or can benefit) from medication? It really depends upon the degree to which you are experiencing the symptoms of MVP. Mild structural MVP, where you have only a systolic click, may not require much aggressive treatment at all, unless you're very concerned and really want to be preventive.

If, in addition to systolic click, you also have a late systolic murmur (indicating mitral regurgitation), this indicates more moderate MVP involvement, possibly requiring more aggressive treatment. Why? There may be a slightly increased risk for endocarditis or progressive mitral regurgitation.

Significant mitral regurgitation suggests more severe MVP. Although the percentage of individuals in this group is very small, these are the individuals who are at the greatest risk for endocarditis or (an even smaller percentage) the need for mitral valve surgery. It is much more common for individuals who are in this category to receive medication as part of their treatment.

Many of the typical symptoms that are associated with MVP are often due to anxiety or an imbalance of the autonomic nervous system. They often respond to medication—for example, beta blockers that can help to control the adrenal system and the autonomic nervous system. But medication should really only be used when the symptoms are more pronounced and do not respond to nonmedical techniques.

THE ROLE OF MEDICATION

Believe it or not, some people welcome drugs as a powerful way to control problems in the body. Others are afraid of their power, and of eventually becoming dependent on them. Still others resent the presence of any artificial substances in their bodies. Where do your feelings fit in?

It is certainly more desirable to treat MVP without medication. But there may be cases where, regardless of your attitudes toward using medication, your physician may feel that medication is necessary. If so, it is essential that you take it properly. Otherwise it can be very dangerous. Unfortunately, even when medication comes into the treatment program, some symptoms of MVP may still continue to exist. So let's talk about medication. The goal? If you need it, you'll want to be able to cope with it.

There are various kinds of drugs that may be helpful in controlling MVP symptoms. Because of the chemical nature of these drugs and the way they may interact with your body, it is extremely important that you follow your doctor's orders in taking the drugs prescribed for you. Do not play with medications that haven't been prescribed (or, as a matter of fact, even with the ones that have been prescribed)!

WHAT TO TAKE

How is it determined which medication is going to be used? In prescribing a drug program, your physician will take into consideration the severity of your condition at the time, as well as the symptoms you're experiencing. Also considered are any other drugs you may be taking, your age, and your overall health, among other factors. But even when all these factors are taken into consideration, doctors are still not sure exactly how a certain medication is going to affect you. So in many cases, trial-and-error is necessary in order to determine the proper dosage. You may need to try different kinds of medication for periods of time in order to arrive at the combination that can best help you. This may be very frustrating, but the results can be worthwhile. Make sure you understand exactly why you're taking any medication and what it's supposed to do.

HOW AND WHEN TO TAKE MEDICATION

Besides knowing what medication you're taking and why you're taking it, you should completely understand when to take it and how. For example, certain medications should be taken after meals. Others may be taken during a meal. Still others may have to be taken on an empty stomach. Some medication should be taken with water, some with food, and some in other ways.

So far, you know the "what" (which medication you are taking), "why" you are taking it, "when" to take it, and "how." But you also need to know "how much" to take and "how often" to take it. (It seems like "where" to take your medication is really the only thing that's left up to you!) The "how much" and "how often," of course, will be supplied by your physician, but you'll still want to understand the answers.

Each person has different needs as far as dose and frequency are concerned. What somebody else takes, even if this person seems to have the same problem, may not necessarily be appropriate for you. The dosage and the frequency of the medication also can be based on the reaction you have to it, how well it's doing what it's supposed to do, and the severity of the problem that is being treated.

Once you begin taking medication in certain dosages, don't attempt to change these dosages on your own. While some medications may be necessary only for a short time, you may need other medication for longer periods of time. Whatever the duration, recognize that your medication is being prescribed to help you.

You probably want to take as little medication as possible. Very few physicians will keep you on high doses of any medication unless they feel it's absolutely essential. If you're taking a substantial dose of any drug, then there must be a reason for it. Don't be afraid to ask your doctor about it. Every good doctor should be able and willing to explain prescribed medication and why you need it. If you're feeling good and you feel like you need less medication, consult your physician first. Then you can plan out a program for reducing medication with your physician.

THEY JUST DON'T GET ALONG

Don't attempt to take any medications other than those prescribed for you. Check with your physician to see if any other medications are appropriate. If you need to take many different pills, it's important that you not play with your dosage, play with the times you take the pills, or move around the number of pills you take at a particular time. Follow your doctor's prescription as carefully as possible.

If you go to other physicians, there could be a problem if they prescribe medications that absolutely should not be taken with your MVP medications. The advantage to having one main physician is obvious. Any other doctor that you may need can then consult with your primary physician to make sure treatment strategies will work together and won't make you worse. Because certain medications are chemically incompatible, you should never mix drugs without knowing the combination is safe. Don't take the chance. Check it out.

SIDE EFFECTS

One of the reasons you might not like the idea of being on medication is that you may be concerned about what the medication may do to your body, or what the side effects may be. Side effects are the "less than pleasant" consequences that indicate that a drug is interacting with your body in a way other than the one that was intended. This is probably one of the biggest concerns about medication. Because medication causes chemical changes within the body, side effects may occur whenever medication is taken. Unfortunately, the more powerful the drug, the more potent the side effects. However, here's an interesting thought. Although no one really loves the thought of experiencing side effects from a particular medication, at least the side effects show you that the drug is potent. It's working! Hopefully, it will have an impact on the symptoms it is trying to alleviate. So remember that the benefits for your body are usually much more important than any potential side effects. Otherwise, your doctor wouldn't prescribe the medication! Physicians are aware of possible side effects, and they won't prescribe any medication that's not necessary (or at higher dosages than are necessary). If side effects do have a particularly harsh impact on you, then your physician may have to weigh the advantages against the disadvantages.

With any drug, it is important to find the lowest dosage that could possibly be effective in helping the person. This is the way to maximize the productivity of the medication and still hopefully minimize any potential side effects.

Minimizing side effects is one reason why it's important to take medication exactly the way it's been prescribed for you. Also, you should report any medication difficulties you experience to your physician.

GETTING DOWN TO SPECIFICS

Let's talk about some of the medications that can be helpful in treating mitral valve prolapse. They can be divided into five categories:

- Beta Blockers
- Calcium Channel Blockers
- Antianxiety Medications
- Antidepressant Medications
- Miscellaneous Drugs

Let's discuss these categories in a little more detail.

Beta Blockers

Beta blockers, also called beta-adrenergic blocking agents, are the most commonly used medications for MVP. These drugs are often used to lower blood pressure and slow the heart rate. If you have palpitations, you may benefit from beta blockers.

Why are they called "beta blockers"? Apparently, they act on a specific type of cell structure, commonly found in the blood vessels and the heart. This cell is called a beta cell receptor.

Although beta blockers are most often thought of as heart drugs, they do have other uses. With individuals who have MVP, they may be helpful in reducing chest pain and controlling blood pressure, migraines, and rapid heartbeat. If it is determined that you're experiencing arrhythmias and they need to be treated with medication, beta blockers may be used.

However, because any of the medications that may be used for arrhythmia problems have to be taken daily and may have occasional side effects, it would be better, especially if the MVP symptoms are mild, that they not be used. For example, beta blockers may be helpful in controlling palpitations, but they may cause more fatigue problems.

Examples of beta blockers commonly used are Inderal, Tenormin, and Lopressor.

Calcium Channel Blockers

Although it's still not exactly understood how these drugs work, calcium channel blockers are occasionally used in helping those with MVP. Some believe these drugs help to dilate the arteries. This can help to reduce spasms in the arteries, as well as lowering blood pressure. It also seems that individuals who take calcium channel blockers are better able to tolerate exercise. Some people who take these drugs report reductions in both fatigue and chest pain as a result.

Among the side effects occasionally reported with calcium channel blockers are significantly low blood pressure, reduced heart rate, and peripheral edema (buildup of fluids).

Examples of calcium channel blockers are Procardia, Cardizem, and Isoptin.

Antianxiety Medications

Much attention is given to the anxiety and panic that so often accompany the structural problems of MVP. Many people are able to reduce these symptoms through nonpharmacological methods (such as relaxation techniques, exercise, and other stress management strategies). But if your doctor feels that medication would be helpful, especially if you've been experiencing panic attacks, there are three subcategories of medications that may be helpful.

The first subcategory of such drugs is the benzodiazapines. These include drugs such as Xanax and Klonopin, which have been effective in helping some people deal with panic. These medications are similar to other popular drugs, such as Valium and Librium, and are all able to control anxiety. But Valium and Librium are not considered panic attack medications.

The drugs in this subcategory are easy to take and usually have relatively few side effects. The main problem with them is that they may become habit forming.

The second subcategory of drugs that may be helpful for dealing with panic attacks is the tricyclic antidepressants. These medications were actually among the earliest ones to be effective in dealing with panic, but they are not used as often any more, since more effective medications have been found. Two of the drugs that may be found in this category are Tofranil and Norpramin.

The third subcategory of drugs is the MAO inhibitors. Some consider this group of drugs to be most effective as panic-controlling drugs. However, they probably require the most rigid compliance of the three groups, in order to minimize any side effects that may occur. For example, if you're taking an MAO inhibitor, it is very important not to take any medications such as antihistamines or decongestants, which might be incompatible and cause further problems. Examples of drugs found in this category are Nardil and Parnate.

In using any of these medications for panic attacks, keep in mind that these medications, even if they are effective, are really effective only in blocking panic attacks, not curing them. It is still important that you deal with any specific triggers for the panic attacks and implement the changes necessary to resolve them.

Antidepressant Medications

Because depression can unfortunately be common for many people with MVP, it has been included in this chapter. There are many different antidepressants, including the tricyclics and MAO inhibitors mentioned in the previous section. They work in different ways, and result in different possible side effects. To benefit best from this category of medication, you should get the latest information from your physician, or a psychiatrist recommended by your physician.

Examples of antidepressants include Desyrel, Elavil, Ludiomil, Pamelor, Prozac, and Sinequan.

Miscellaneous Drugs

There are many other types of drugs that may be helpful for individuals with MVP. For example, because migraine headaches may be an unpleasant symptom, antimigraine drugs may be helpful. Medication may be necessary for allergies, or to control water retention. Autonomic nervous system problems may respond to certain types of medications. There are so many possible combinations of drugs that may be helpful that it may take time to determine the "formula" that's best for you. But that's why working with your doctor is so important.

Preventive Medication

Any discussion of medication for MVP would not be complete without mentioning the preventive use of medication. Some doctors advise many of their patients who have MVP to take antibiotics, such as amoxicillin, before dental or surgical procedures. This is called antibiotic prophylaxis. Some doctors believe in this very strongly, while others do not.

Why are antibiotics sometimes helpful? An excessive number of bacteria may be released into the bloodstream when dental or other surgical procedures are done. In a small number of cases, more likely when mitral regurgitation keeps the blood from flowing properly, this bacteria may come to rest on the mitral valve. If the bacteria grows, endocarditis, an infection that can affect the mitral valve, may result. Although this does not happen very often at all, if it does it could prove to be quite serious. So there are some physicians who believe that the best course of action is a preventive one. They suggest using antibiotics to "be ready for the bacteria" before these procedures are even done.

What determines whether or not you should undergo antibiotic prophylaxis? Most doctors believe that it usually depends on how pronounced your prolapse is, and what degree of blood regurgitation you're experiencing. Most experts believe that antiobiotic prophylaxis is necessary if you have mitral regurgitation as evidenced by a murmur. But it does not seem to be as necessary if you just show signs of systolic clicks or if your MVP is silent (meaning that if, when listening with a stethoscope, doctors don't hear any clicks or murmurs). This is certainly something to discuss with your physician, so that you're reassured as to what the best course of action is for you.

But, you might ask, if antibiotic prophylaxis reduces the chances of infective endocarditis, why doesn't everyone use it? Well, one of the reasons is that some doctors are afraid that some patients may react negatively to the antibiotics. They believe that if you're going to have negative reactions to the antibiotics, then you're better off taking your chances without them. For example, if you're allergic to penicillin, you shouldn't be on penicillin! Others feel that if you don't have any negative reactions to the antibiotics, you'd be better off taking them if you are going to have dental work done. Remember that each individual case is different and it is important to check with your physician to know exactly what is best for you.

CAUTIONS!

Not all drugs are good for you, even if they're good drugs. By working closely with your physician, you're helping to make sure that all medications you take are appropriate for you. There are certain drugs (and especially over-the-counter medications) you should not use because of the possibility of aggravating the symptoms of MVP. It is suggested that you should not take medications that contain caffeine, epinephrine, ephedrine, or pseudoephedrine. Examples of medications containing these ingredients include Fiorinal, Darvon, Anacin, Dexatrim, Midol, and Vanquish (which contain caffeine); or Contac, Robitussin, and Sudafed (which contain pseudoephedrine). You've heard this a lot already, but: Work with your doctor! Question, learn, and help yourself. Check with your physician before taking even the most innocent-seeming over-the-counter drug. You never know when you might have a bad reaction.

You also have to be careful about any bad mixes. For example, tranquilizers should never be taken at the same time as alcohol. There are plenty of other such cautions. Please don't hesitate to ask questions. Many of these incompatibilities could have extremely dangerous outcomes, either by making your symptoms worse, by interfering with the desired benefits of the drugs you're taking, or by causing additional problems.

Working With Your Pharmacist

It is almost impossible for any physician to keep up with all the thousands of different types of prescription drugs on the market. However, this is the pharmacist's specialty. Frequently, pharmacists know even more than physicians as far as what drugs can go together and what drugs interact dangerously.

So it can be very helpful for you to develop a good working relationship with your local pharmacist. Not only will your pharmacist be able to tell you about the medication that has been prescribed for you, but he or she may be able to help you reduce costs. Occasionally, generic products may be available that cost less than brand-name products. However, in some individuals, the generic drug will not work as well as the brand-name medication. If you have a good relationship with your pharmacist, you will find it a lot easier to get the medication you need.

You may find that dealing with the same drugstore and pharmacist is very comforting. The more time you spend there, the better the pharmacist will get to know you and your specific needs. You'll have somebody else looking out for your welfare in addition to your physician!

What happens if you go into a pharmacy with a prescription and the pharmacist suggests substituting another drug (or a generic one) for the medication that was originally prescribed for you? There may be nothing wrong with this, but make sure you consult your physician before making such a substitution. Of course, if your physician prescribes generically, the pharmacist can decide.

ADDITIONAL MEDICATION 'MINDERS

Once you've begun taking medication, make sure you let your physician know how effective the drugs are in helping you with your condition. Any significant changes in your health, whether good or bad, should be reported to your physician. In this way, your doctor will be best able to decide whether or not to keep prescribing the medication you're taking.

As with most categories of drugs, there are a number of specific brands in each category. Although they generally work the same way, there are some minor differences between the drugs. Why is this important? If, for some reason, you're not able to take one without side effects, you might be able to do well on another drug in the same category. Your doctor will work with you on this.

Keep a list in your wallet of the medications you take. Show the list to your doctor, or pharmacist, or anyone else who needs to know what you're taking. (Makes for great "show and tell" at the P.T.A. meetings!)

You may experience certain emotional reactions to taking medication (such as depression or anger). This must be dealt with. (If necessary, look back at the chapters on coping with your emotions.) Remember: If it's really necessary for you to take medication, you might as well let it do what it's supposed to. Accept it and don't let it bother you.

A FINAL PRESCRIPTION

This chapter doesn't include all medications used by people with mitral valve prolapse. Instead, it emphasizes some of the more common ones. But at least this information will give you an idea of what's important to know in order to better deal with medication. So if your doctor prescribes something new, ask about it. Not only will you probably feel better physically, but you'll know why!

20

Surgery

Mitral valve replacement is still considered to be an acceptable procedure in those comparatively rare and extreme cases where it is necessary. It is used more often in older individuals who have had MVP for longer periods of time. It is a comparatively safe procedure, with a very low mortality rate, even though it is open-heart surgery. It usually does clear up the problems that may result from mitral regurgitation.

Not too many people cherish the thought of "going under the knife." In the past, surgery replacing the mitral valve was rarely considered unless it was a last resort. Since 1962, surgery has been successful in many cases in which the valve was damaged beyond repair. So let's discuss surgery as a treatment for MVP.

WHEN IS SURGERY CONSIDERED?

A very small percentage of people with MVP may, in time, require heart valve replacement surgery. The main reason that some people with MVP have required valve surgery is that they had progressive valvular incompetence (in other words, their valves just were not working effectively), and the damage caused by this incompetence was becoming dangerous. There are usually only a small percentage of people with MVP who have a severe valve problem. In general, for most people with MVP, this does not happen.

VALVE REPLACEMENT OR RECONSTRUCTION

Ever since surgery was first used for MVP, there have been disagreements as to whether the valve should be replaced or reconstructed. There are two main factors that are most often involved in deciding which is best. The first involves the degree of damage to the valve (a severely damaged valve may not be reconstructable). And the second is that reconstructed valves may eliminate rejection as a potential problem. (Artificial valve replacements may, like any other foreign body, be rejected by the immune system, although this isn't much of a problem since the valves are often inert plastics or metals.)

PROBLEMS WITH SURGERY

There are a number of potential problems with valve surgery in general. First of all, the cost can be considerable. But for somebody whose ineffective valve is dangerous, the cost is a very minor consideration! There are other risks, as there would be with any major heart surgery. These risks involve factors such as your age, physical condition, other diseases (such as hypertension, diabetes, or other coronary artery disease), and how much heart damage has already occurred as a result of the valve problem. The pros and cons of surgery must take into consideration all of these risks.

In addition, there are potential risks following surgery that must be considered. For example, if an artificial valve is implanted, it has none of the normal germ-killing properties that normal healthy tissue has. As a result, bacteria may form on the surface of this new valve. This may eventually affect the lining of the heart, and may need to be dealt with by using antibiotic therapy.

Another potential risk following surgery is the possibility of blood clots. As a result, individuals who have had valve replacement surgery are usually required to take blood-thinner anticoagulant medication, possibly for the rest of their lives.

Despite the fact that these problems need to be considered, if valve damage is such that there is no alternative, these considerations are minor, indeed.

However, even though surgery can't cure all of these symptoms, at least it can significantly relieve many of the problems related to the structural defect. For example, a primary goal is to stop blood regurgitation. Surgery will replace or repair the defective mitral valve. However, it will not improve the problems resulting from an imbalance in the autonomic nervous system.

THINGS TO THINK ABOUT

There are some important things for you to think about if surgery is a possibility for you.

- Get a second opinion. This is always important before deciding whether or not surgery is the treatment for you.

- Ask your primary physician for recommendations regarding which cardiovascular surgeon should perform the surgery.

- If you do have valve replacement surgery, it probably will be necessary for you to be on anticoagulants or blood thinners for the rest of your life. There are other risks involved following surgery. There have been cases where individuals having valve replacement surgery experienced stroke or hemorrhage.

- Discuss what's involved in the operation and what kind of rehabilitation will follow. What will you need to know before, during, and after the procedure? Feel free to ask questions. Remember: Preparation for surgery makes the outcome better (and easier)!

21

Activities

What to do, what to do? Sure you have mitral valve prolapse, but what does this mean in terms of the basic activities in your life? What can you do and what can't you do? Even if you feel wonderful, you'll probably feel nervous about participating in any vigorous activities. You may want to minimize the strain you put on your body. In fact, you may not even have the strength!

Each person is different. The kinds of things you did before being diagnosed with MVP can influence what you can or want to do now. Your current physical condition is also a determining factor. If you've been experiencing a lot of chest pain, for example, you may not want to expend a lot of energy until your doctor has given you the green light (or even a cautious yellow) to resume. So let's discuss some of the more important types of activities that people participate in.

WORKING

Working can be very important for you. Besides its being an important source of your income (can't overlook that!), working can help you feel like your life is proceeding as usual. You may be concerned (an understatement!) if you feel that MVP may threaten the possibility of your working. This may interfere with your financial security.

Even though you have mitral valve prolapse, you'll probably want to do as much of what you used to as possible. Are you afraid that you'll feel like less of a person if you have to stop working? Work is important. It helps you to feel independent. It gives you a sense of self-fulfillment. It provides more financial strength than not working, of course. And it provides an important component of your social life.

Many people question whether or not they should work. The answer is: If you want to, and you need to, and you can, then you should! But you may have to make some modifications because you don't want to take a chance of running yourself down.

Stamina Shortage

You may be concerned that symptoms of MVP may interfere with your being able to perform adequately on the job. Mitral valve prolapse may cause you to experience fatigue or other discomfort. This may affect your work productivity, especially if your treatment is not controlling your symptoms as well as you'd like it to. Your work rate may slow down, you may be absent or late more often, and you simply may not feel physically able to work. You may get tired easily and feel that you just don't have the stamina necessary to complete your job satisfactorily. If your employer is aware of any of these problems, you may be afraid that your job will be in jeopardy. You may fear that your value to the company may decrease.

What can you do? Build up your stamina slowly. Don't expect too much at once. Pacing yourself is probably the most important thing you can do. Take rest breaks whenever necessary (and possible) to "recharge your batteries." If you're not sure how much you can do, do what you can and let your body be your guide.

Bending the Rules?

Employers are not required by law to make any special provisions for you because you have mitral valve prolapse. You still have to do what you're supposed to do. However, if you're an important employee, your company probably will want to retain your services. You may be able to continue working at a particular job with only a few modifications (such as changing your chair, desk, location, or a few of the activities you used to do). Changing your hours also may be helpful.

You may be uncomfortable about approaching your employer to find out if these changes can be made. It may bother you to seek special treatment on your job, but this is something you may have to do. These changes may be small in comparison to the problems your company might face if they had to hire a new employee to replace you.

You may fear that you'll have difficulty with other employees if you receive special treatment. This may not be true at all, but your anticipation or apprehension of this happening may cause problems.

Lack of Understanding

Darlene had been working in the same office for eight years. Because of MVP, she had been having more difficulty completing her tasks and getting to work each day. Unfortunately, her supervisor was a demanding perfectionist who apparently was not willing to bend at all for Darlene. He called her in for review and made it perfectly clear that unless her performance and attendance improved, she would be out of a job. In addition to calling her in, he frequently reminded her (in both subtle and blunt ways) that he was watching her. The pressure on Darlene became so hard to bear that it began to affect her emotional and physical health. What do you do if you feel you're being harassed?

Your employer may express displeasure about curtailed work time. What if an ultimatum is given, stating that if productivity does not improve, you will be discharged (polite, aren't I?)? This is another potential problem. So what do you do? You do the best you can. If an employer doesn't understand enough about mitral valve prolapse to know that you must pace yourself, and shows little or no willingness to cooperate, then you're probably better off not continuing employment there. You don't want to look for more trouble.

Changing Jobs

How appropriate is it to discuss with an employer the medical condition itself? As with many medical diseases or conditions, there are some employers who would be very supportive and understanding, and there are others who would be somewhat apprehensive about hiring or retaining an individual who has any kind of heart problem. (Remember, even though MVP is not considered to be a serious heart problem, and employers should not be concerned about it, they may not know that!) The reality is that most people with MVP are able to fulfill work obligations much the same as anybody else. So it would be necessary for information about MVP to be provided to those people in decision-making capacities. Hopefully, they'll recognize that MVP should not interfere with job hiring or retaining decisions.

Don't stay at a job if it's not right for you. Consider transferring to another one or getting additional training to move into a new job. In some cases, individuals with certain job experiences and backgrounds are unable to work in jobs for which they were trained because of their new condition. For example, Lenny (a thirty-nine-year-old father of two) had been working in construction. But doctors felt he shouldn't continue this type of work because it was too strenuous for him. Lenny became very depressed. He didn't know what else he could do. He shut down emotionally, rather than face the prospect of not being able to work. He was even afraid that he didn't have the ability to go out and get new training.

How do you deal with this? One way might be to check with any of the government-provided services that offer vocational counseling. Counselors in these offices will work with you to determine exactly what your aptitude is for different jobs. You can then get training and support to help you obtain employment in the fields you're interested in. If you need help in finding jobs that are appropriate for you, you may want to check with the state employment services. These services are available free of charge and have specialists that can help you to find jobs that are suitable for your needs.

For financial reasons, should you wait until your employment is terminated? This has its pros and cons. If you receive unemployment benefits for losing your job, this could ease financial burdens. But if subsequent employers are reluctant to hire you because of the grounds for dismissal, is it worth it? Only you can decide, and you'll probably have to base your decision on your own unique situation. It's a very important question, since your psychological state is so important in your coping with mitral valve prolapse. If your employment is aggravating you, then changes may have to be made.

Is Working Your Only Option?

What are the advantages of working? Some of the benefits are satisfaction, productivity, money, and pride. But a paying job is not the only type of satisfying work. There are plenty of other meaningful, productive activities that can be done voluntarily. Check with non-profit organizations, hospitals, schools, senior citizen centers, and the like. They can always use some extra help. You'll feel good about yourself, too. Volunteers also can work with religious, political, or charitable organizations.

What if you just don't want to work? Some individuals with MVP are happy if they choose not to work. But don't use your condition as an excuse for not working. This may indicate that something else is bothering you. You may want to explore that further.

SCHOOL

For school-age children with MVP, school problems can be similar to work-related problems. Attendance may decrease because there may be times when the child just doesn't feel physically up to going. The child may be concerned about going to school because of the reduced number of activities that can be participated in because of physical restrictions. A child with mitral valve prolapse also might be concerned about reactions from other students while in school. Teachers should be informed so that they will be aware of these potential problems.

RECREATION

People with mitral valve prolapse may still be able to participate in a number of different types of activity including boating, skating, golf, tennis, and dancing. Whether or not you do depends on your condition. If your doctor has given you the green light, and you try an activity without experiencing excessive fatigue, pain, shortness of breath, or other problems, you're probably okay. On the other hand, there may be times when your condition keeps you from feeling like you can do it. However, if your doctor approves, at least you know that you can try. It's up to you and your doctor to decide which activities are best for you.

Why is it so helpful to participate in activities that you enjoy? They can help improve your ability to take care of yourself. They can help promote and maintain your participation in the normal activities of daily living, and they can certainly provide you with benefits in both the social and psychological aspects of your life.

ACTIVITIES OF DAILY LIVING

Among the things you do each day are the normal, routine tasks known as the activities of daily living (ADL). But there's a problem. Any restrictions you're experiencing from mitral valve prolapse may limit these activities. This can be frustrating. Why? Probably because, prior to being diagnosed, you may have taken such simple tasks for granted. The way you're feeling now, however, may make you depressed and upset, rather than enthusiastic about trying to conquer the problem.

What if you can't do what you want to do? You may not want to ask for help. You may feel that it takes away some of your dignity. This can make you very uncomfortable. However, the future can be brighter! In a very short period of time, you can reorganize your lifestyle, your house, and your daily activities in a way that can reduce your difficulties and salvage a lot of your dignity. Remember: Not all people with mitral valve prolapse experience these problems. (And if you do, doesn't it make sense to see what you can do to improve the situation?)

Modifying your lifestyle or your home is not the same as giving in to MVP. However, it may be an important part of helping you to learn to live most effectively and cope most successfully with your condition.

Easing the Load

Your goal is to make daily living as easy as possible. Why? An important part of living with MVP is learning to conserve energy. So you'll want to reduce or eliminate those activities that aren't necessary and simplify those that are! Conserving your energy can be very important in helping you to avoid much of the excessive fatigue that can be a negative factor in living with MVP.

In many cases, problems with daily living can be conquered without professional help. It can be very satisfying for you to develop your own solutions to these problems. This can be one of the most important ways of coping with MVP. Of course, any questions you have can be bounced off physicians, physical therapists, or other health professionals.

Start by trying to evaluate everything you do on a day-to-day basis and seeing how you can make every single thing you do easier. Realistically, you know you cannot eliminate all the activities that you need to do around your home. However, what's wrong with finding easier ways of doing them? Is this taking the lazy way out? Of course not. You are simply recognizing that every bit of energy you save from one activity will give you more energy to do something else.

Any specific suggestions? There are lots of things you can do to help yourself with daily living. For example, you'll want to learn how to moderate your activities. Plan them out carefully and pace yourself. One thing you may find helpful is to chart out your activities, including required activities as well as social and leisure activities. This may help you to become better organized so that you can pace yourself more effectively.

Try to plan activities in advance so you can figure out exactly how you're going to do them, what equipment you're going to need, and how much time you can spend doing them before you may need to rest. This will help you to reduce the amount of strain, both physically and emotionally, and will keep you from getting overtired.

Try to reduce the amount of energy you expend in performing any activities. If necessary, modify the method that you use. Eliminate any unnecessary activity. Rest intermittently and whenever needed. You'll then be able to do more of what you want or need to do. And you'll accomplish it in a healthier way.

Any activities that may make you physically uncomfortable should be modified as much as possible. And you certainly don't want to do things that cause pain, even if the pain is of very short duration. You may want to reorganize your home and your habits in such a way that makes movement easier and puts things within easy reach. You can lubricate drawers so that they open and close more easily. You can wear clothing that is easier to get on and off. There are also a number of different types of gadgets that may make life easier for you.

TRAVELING

Since you were diagnosed with mitral valve prolapse, have you been afraid that the condition would interfere with travel plans? Some people are concerned about traveling with MVP. Need it be this way?

Definitely not. Very few restrictions need to be placed on your travel plans. As a matter of fact, you probably can go just about anywhere!

Sure, there may be some individuals with mitral valve prolapse who avoid traveling. But their concerns may have nothing to do with MVP. Some don't travel simply because they feel it's too expensive. Or others may not even like to travel. But plenty of others with MVP do travel, whether their trips are short or long. Some travel simply to prove to themselves that they can. This doesn't mean that there are no fears attached. But they do want to prove to themselves that they can do it, and that traveling, as one of life's pleasures, is possible.

As with any other aspect of living with your MVP, planning ahead and taking the proper precautions can allow you to travel with a free mind (although not with free airfare!). What types of planning ahead should you do before a vacation? Let's explore some of them.

What are the symptoms you are experiencing? Do what you can to adequately prepare to cope with these symptoms. For example, some people experience certain symptoms of MVP syndrome, either before they're traveling or during their trip. This may be because of anticipation of flying, which can create anxiety or panic, and has nothing to do with MVP! If you experience anxiety or panic related to flying there are a number of things to consider. You might decide to go on a different type of vacation. Or, you might want to use some of the more reasonable methods or medications that can be helpful in dealing with these concerns. If, on the other hand, the problems you are experiencing are not panic-based, but rather are symptoms such as shortness of breath or tachycardia, there are other things to try. Drink plenty of fluids. Eliminate any caffeine or sugar. Work on your relaxation. This may help to stabilize the situation. Other than that, travel and enjoy.

If you think you might like to travel, discuss it with your physician first. Chances are, if you're able to get around your own neighborhood without assistance, you probably can handle traveling with confidence. Your doctor will let you know if any MVP-related symptoms indicate a need to restrict travelling.

If you do plan a trip, it's always a good idea to take out trip-cancellation insurance, especially if you stand to lose a lot of money because of last-minute, non-refundable cancellations. If getting around is a problem, you may opt to use wheelchairs to reduce fatigue as well as to increase the distance you can travel. That might not be a bad idea. But some people are afraid of being seen in a wheelchair, or are even more afraid that once they use them, they'll be stuck in them forever. Neither of these fears is valid, but both can interfere with happy travel plans. Work on them.

When making hotel reservations or other accommodations, make sure that they fit your needs. You'll want to know where you can get proper medical care if necessary. So prepare for this. Write out a list of clinics, hospitals, and physicians in different parts of the world where you may be traveling.

Taking Medication and Other Supplies

One of your biggest concerns about traveling may be: What happens if I run out of sufficient medication or other supplies? There are two things you can do. First, have extra medication and supplies packed in case any unexpected situations arise. Second, ask your physician to write up extra prescriptions to take with you. At least you'll be prepared if you need more. You also may want to ask if you can keep your doctor "on call" so that you can contact him or her in an emergency. If you're going to a foreign country, you may want the prescription translated into the language of that country in case the pharmacist has difficulty understanding English.

If you're flying, carry all medications and other necessary supplies with you. Do not pack all supplies in your luggage. Why? If your luggage ends up in Phoenix when you're flying to Chicago, you don't want to be left without what you need. Besides, if for any reason you need a pill during the flight, it would be rather inconsiderate of you to ask the flight attendant to climb down into the baggage hold to get it!

Identify Yourself

It's always a good idea to travel with complete identification, not just for your luggage but for yourself. The Medic Alert bracelet is accepted worldwide as identification of a person with a medical problem. Although some people might not see a need for identification bracelets for MVP (or may be embarrassed if it brings extra attention), it is a good idea if you're on medication, or if you have other medical conditions. And don't worry about extra attention. The bracelets are usually attractive, and most people will glance at them only casually, if at all.

If you do decide to wear such a bracelet, you'll keep in your wallet an identification card with complete details about your condition, any medication you need, and any other pertinent information. Again, if you're going to a foreign country, you might make sure that this information is translated into the language of that country. What if foreign languages were never your forte? Try checking with a teacher of that particular foreign language in a local school. Check with the airline that flies to that country. Representatives who speak the language probably would be willing to translate for you. As a last resort, you may want to check with the foreign embassy of that particular country. This may take a little extra time, but your mind will be more at ease when you do travel.

To Confirm . . .

Remember, many individuals with MVP feel absolutely no reluctance to travel anywhere. If you haven't traveled recently, you may want to build up your confidence by taking short trips first. Taking a three-month trip around the world might be a bit much! Even an overnight trip might be traumatic. Start with a couple of day trips, then weekend trips, working your way up to short-distance, week-long excursions. Expanding your travel activities slowly is a good way to develop your confidence. So enjoy a wonderful vacation. Don't forget to send me a postcard.

A FINAL EXERTION

Keeping active is a very important part of coping with mitral valve prolapse. You want to feel productive and enjoy life. You don't want to let MVP confine you to your closet. So don't let it. Do what you physically can, but do!

22

Financial Problems

Having MVP can be a pain in the pocketbook! Any chronic medical condition can be expensive, and mitral valve prolapse is no exception.

Why are the financial costs so high? The cost of treatment, doctor's visits, and other medical costs, as well as the cost of medication, hospitalization (if needed), and laboratory tests, all add up. In addition, money is lost from any work days that are missed because of symptoms. The cost (and source) for each person with MVP varies considerably. But it may not take long for financial security to drain into a financial problem.

INSURANCE CAN BE AN ASSURANCE

Fortunately, some people can have some of their costs defrayed by insurance. Insurance coverage is essential. For individuals with mitral valve prolapse, certain costs may be reimbursable by third-party payments. Insurance companies do cover a number of medical costs. But what happens if you run out of money or insurance, or if your coverage is not good enough? Because you have a chronic medical condition, you may have more difficulty getting either life or health insurance. Speak to a reputable insurance agent and find out exactly what you are entitled to.

WORK OR HOME

Financial problems arise from lost earnings or income. You may not be working at all, or perhaps you'll only be working at a part-time job. Your condition may affect your ability to work. This may cause problems with your job. So it's possible that your "employability" will be reduced because of your MVP.

Mitral valve prolapse also can be costly because of changes at home. You may need additional help around the house, such as a baby-sitter or a cleaning person. These things cost money, adding to your financial burden. As medical costs rise, your budget can become tighter and tighter. If costs continue to skyrocket, you may feel like you're being strangled!

CAN ANYTHING HELP?

Mitral valve prolapse need not be alarmingly expensive if you're careful. If you take proper care of yourself and follow your treatment correctly, hopefully you'll control the condition sufficiently and you can keep costs down.

If you require medication, the use of generic drugs can save you money. Generic medication is sold by its chemical name rather than a more common brand name. Ask your physician if it's acceptable to take generic medication. (Remember, not all generics work as well as brand name medication.)

If medical costs are overwhelming you, consider attending a clinic. Because clinics usually operate on a sliding-scale fee schedule, you may be able to get quality medical care at a reduced cost. In some cases, you may even see the same physician you'd normally see, since many physicians graciously donate their time to clinics.

If you have questions about financial problems, you may want to check with local agencies such as the Department of Social Services, or organizations such as the American Heart Association. They may be able to provide you with information and resources. They can tell you which benefits you may be qualified for and how to apply for them.

So before you do anything, talk to people. Find out what others have done. How do you find them? Ask your physician or other health professionals for suggestions, or contact other organizations in your community for ideas. Speak to others in similar situations to find out how they handle their financial problems. Even though you may initially be embarrassed to bring up the subject, the common bond that exists among people with medically-induced financial problems tends to smooth this over rather quickly. You'll be glad you brought it up!

GOVERNMENT PROGRAMS MAY OR MAY NOT HELP

Some government insurance programs may be important sources of financial support. Individuals with a wide variety of medical problems may be covered (at least to some degree) by Medicare, where eligibility is determined by age, chronic disability, or both; Medicaid, where benefits vary from state to state; or social security disability insurance. Unfortunately, mitral valve prolapse may not be reimbursable under these programs unless there are other underlying conditions that qualify. The best thing to do is to speak to health professionals, check with the appropriate agencies, or call the American Heart Association and ask for advice regarding whom you should contact.

PART IV
Interacting With Other People

23

Coping With Others—
An Introduction

You do not live your life alone (unless you're reading this book on a deserted island in the Pacific). You interact with many people every day. So you'll certainly want to be able to deal with any difficulties in interpersonal relationships. For example, what are others going to think? How are they going to react? Are they going to ask questions? What kinds of answers will they listen to and what kinds will turn them away? These are some of the questions that may bother you.

Since you'll probably be with other people during a good part of your waking hours, it makes sense to be aware of how MVP may affect these relationships. Obviously, different problems can exist in different relationships. But before we begin discussing each type of relationship specifically, there are a few general points to be made.

DO UNTO OTHERS . . .

When you interact with others, you don't want to become too wrapped up in your own feelings. If you disregard the feelings of others, you'll also prevent others from getting close to you. Consider how others feel, just as you'd like them to consider your feelings. What does this mean? You're not the only one who has to cope with MVP. Important people in your life also may be having a hard time, simply because you mean a lot to them. Remember that. Some people tend to feel that their problems don't affect anyone else. You might think, "How can they feel upset? It's happening to me!" But is that fair? Take your family, for example. A problem for you is also a problem for them. Of course, it may be affecting you differently. Maybe you're the one experiencing the restrictions and the physical changes, as well as the apprehensions and anxieties, but your condition still affects those who care about you. They don't like to see you suffer. You'll be better able to cope with these important people, as well as help yourself cope better, by remembering this.

YOU CAN'T CHANGE OTHERS

Do you feel that if you try hard enough you can change the attitudes, feelings, or behaviors of others? It doesn't happen that way. Whether they accept your MVP or deny that you have any problem at all, you can't change them. You can only change yourself. Spend more time working on you, and worry less about others. They may change, but it will more likely be as a result of the changes they see in you. Help yourself. Be your own best friend.

LOOK THROUGH THE EYES OF OTHERS

If you have an argument with someone, you may believe that you're right and the other person is wrong. In this case, nothing will be resolved. Try "eyeballing." Take a moment and look at the situation through the eyes of the other person. What does he or she see? What might the other point of view be? This will definitely help you to better understand the problem.

   If you look at the problem only through your own eyes, someone else's behavior may drive you crazy. Looking through the eyes of others can help you to better understand them and to improve your relationship with them. If you then try to have a discussion, this also will help you to explain how you feel.

PRIDE, YES! REVENGE, NO!

Revenge! There are times when you might think, "I only wish that so-and-so could know what it's like to live with the symptoms of mitral valve prolapse for an hour, a day, or a week, so that he/she could understand what I've been going through." But you know this isn't realistic, and you can't sit around waiting for it to happen. Besides, afterward you might not be too pleased with yourself for having such vengeful thoughts. So what should you do? Take pride in yourself. Concentrate on doing what's best for you. If you have to be a little more self-centered and a little less concerned about what other people think, just accept this as one more way of coping with your condition.

A LITTLE SELFISHNESS IS OKAY

What happens if you're feeling rotten, but others want you to keep doing more and more? In the past, you may have had trouble saying no, because you'd either feel guilty or you didn't want to disappoint someone or hurt their feelings. But now you must curtail your generosity because you really don't feel well. Frequently, you may have to give the appearance of being selfish. But don't take this negatively. As long as you don't abuse it, this selfishness can be positive for you. Do for yourself; think of yourself. You're Number One, and that's the way it must be. If you take care of yourself, then you can be in the best shape to deal with others. The reverse does not hold true. If you are best for others, you may not be best for yourself.

BRING ON THE WORLD

Now that we've started with some general ideas, let's see how mitral valve prolapse can affect the different relationships you have with people. Of course, not every chapter will apply to you. You can either read the chapters that are appropriate for you, or read them all and realize that different kinds of problems do exist in any relationship.

24

Your Family

Blood is thicker than water! Your family can be a critical factor in your successful adjustment to MVP. Why? You're probably with your family more than with anyone else. If you get along well with members of your family, you'll have a solid foundation from which to move toward a triumphant adjustment to your condition.

There are various types of problems that may pop up with different members of your family. So let's discuss how to cope with each specific member.

COPING WITH YOUR SPOUSE

Having MVP can have an effect on your marriage. But this doesn't mean that problems can't be resolved. Through better communication, understanding, and counseling (if necessary), there are very few problems that can't be worked out. Let's discuss some of the ways in which a marriage may feel the impact of mitral valve prolapse.

Social Life Changes

Have you had to cut back on your social activities because of restrictions caused by mitral valve prolapse? You may have to curtail some of the activities that you used to enjoy with your spouse. You just may not be able to do as much. This can be hard to take, especially if you both had active social lives before the onset of your condition. Because your spouse does not have MVP, he or she may feel anger, frustration, or helplessness. If, however, your social life is still on hold even after your condition has stabilized, you'll have to ask yourself if this is due to certain fears or apprehensions. If so, refer to other appropriate chapters (such as "Fears and Anxieties") for suggestions and support.

If Family Responsibilities Must Change . . .

Mitral valve prolapse may create the need for temporary or permanent changes in each family member's responsibilities. This can surely be another potential source of friction between you and your spouse, especially when your spouse receives a heavy share of the load. "Re-assigning" chores to different members of the family can be very difficult for all. Lorraine, a thirty-four-year old mother of three, told her husband that he would have to take over all of the household chores, including cooking, cleaning, and even doing windows. Her two older children would have to do all of the grocery shopping and would have to take turns helping their younger brother with homework, bathing, etc.

Despite the fact that Lorraine's family loved her and was concerned about her health, they were all understandably upset, especially her husband. Since he had difficulty even boiling water, he certainly wasn't too thrilled. How can you change things as smoothly as possible? Make changes gradually. Being able to afford household help would make things easier, of course. But regardless of this, try to avoid overwhelming your spouse. Be realistic in your expectations.

How else can you help your spouse to adjust to greater burdens? Make sure free time is still available for the pleasures of life. It's only when the new responsibilities seem to be all-consuming that serious problems may occur. Look at any changes through the eyes of your spouse. Consider how you'd feel if the situation were reversed. Think how upsetting it would be if you no longer had time for things you enjoyed because of added responsibilities and pressures. Discuss it reasonably, and be gentle.

Denial

What do you do if your spouse simply won't accept the fact that you have mitral valve prolapse? You might hear, "Come on, you look fine. What are you complaining about?" This is tough to swallow. You can try to "educate" your spouse, but don't go overboard. If you're constantly badgering, reminding your spouse of the things that have changed because of MVP, you certainly won't convince someone who has obviously been denying its very existence. Your spouse will not accept your condition until ready to do so. Concentrate on your own feelings. Others' feelings may change, but slowly.

In Sickness and in Health? Sorry!

Unfortunately, some marriages have ended because of a chronic medical problem. Any restrictions resulting from mitral valve prolapse have the potential to drive a wedge into what may have previously been a good marriage. Former feelings of closeness and intimacy may be replaced by the unwelcome feelings of coldness and distance. Some spouses have so much difficulty accepting changes in their relationship that the "magic" seems to be washed right out of the marriage.

But it may not be all your spouse's fault. You may be so apprehensive that you can't enjoy your relationship. Your sensitivity may cause you to be less patient. So marital breakups do occur. But realize that about 50 percent of all marriages end in divorce anyway, even when mitral valve prolapse is not involved!

Statistics aside, what do you do if your spouse is frightened and "wants out"? Your spouse's fear, your own condition, and your fears of abandonment all combine to create a horrible package of anxiety, depression, hopelessness, and panic. This package isn't one you can (or should) handle alone and, at this point, you may not be able to talk to your spouse. You may find communication with your spouse either nonexistent or counterproductive. Get some help. Seeking the aid of a professional or an objective outsider may help to smooth over some of the rough edges. If possible, include your mate. But once again, don't force the issue. It's better for you, at least, to get some counseling. If your marriage does end, outside support will be very helpful in getting you back on your feet emotionally.

What About Money?

Mitral valve prolapse can present added money problems, especially for your spouse. If you are the bread-winner, your spouse may fear the unpleasant role of becoming more responsible for financial aspects of family management. If your spouse is the major income-producer, pressure from the added costs of treatment or medication may be tough. Both you and your spouse will worry about whether all obligations can be met (and continue to be met). Money concerns are frequently a major source of friction in any marriage. Here the problem is just compounded. Sit down, talk it over, and be realistic. Although new strains may arise, these things frequently have a way of working themselves out. Be patient, be communicative, and be positive.

Is Sex Affected?

Another area in which MVP may affect a marital relationship is that of sex. The chapter "Sex and Mitral Valve Prolapse" provides more information on this important subject.

A Marital (Con-) Summation

Coping with your spouse while you have mitral valve prolapse can be difficult and, occasionally, impossible. Any marriage has its ups and downs. It has problems that have to be worked out. Having MVP makes relationships more vulnerable to crises and arguments. Working through MVP-related problems requires much more attention to your spouse's feelings and needs. But it's worth it. If problem spots can be smoothed out, your spouse can really be your best ally in helping you adjust to your condition.

COPING WITH CHILDREN

Children need a lot from their parents. This can surely be frustrating if you're unable to provide as much for them as you'd like. You may not be able to do as much, or help them as much. This does not mean that you don't love them or that you're not a good parent. Because

each person lives differently with MVP, there's no way of predict-
ing how much it will affect you physically (or even emotionally).
It may be hard to acknowledge your shortcomings as a parent. But
think about your children. How much do they know about your
condition? How hard is it for them to deal with this new situation?
Let's see how you can help them.

How Do You Explain MVP to Your Children?

The younger the child, the less of an explanation he or she will need.
Anything that you tell a youngster will have to be explained simply.
With very young children, you might just say, "I don't feel well and
I can't do this. I'd like to, but I can't." Unless you're more noticeably
affected, you may not have to say much of anything.

With older children, explanations can be more detailed. Encourage
their questions. Randy, age twelve, knew her mother had MVP. But
her mother couldn't understand why she rarely asked any questions
about it. Was she keeping unhappy thoughts inside, or had she just
accepted it and didn't feel it was necessary to ask anything? Remember: If your children really don't want to ask you anything, they
won't. But let them know that they can if they want to. Upsetting
thoughts kept inside can be even more destructive.

The questions of older children probably will be more direct and
more specific. Resulting discussions, if handled properly, will not
only be helpful for your children—you'll enjoy them too! You'll also
enjoy the great feeling of closeness that can result.

Fielding Children's Questions

How do you answer questions? This depends on the age of the child,
as well as on how much of an answer the child may be looking for.
The best advice is to provide direct answers to the specific questions.
Don't go into detail, unless your child asks for more information.

Think, for example, about parents talking with their children about
sex. Because of the delicate nature of the subject and the discomfort
or anxiety on the part of the parent, more information than necessary
is usually given. Have you heard the anecdote about the very young
child who walked up to his mother and asked, "Mommy, where did
I come from???" The mother started trembling because this was the

first time she had heard such a question from her child. But she nervously explained the various parts of the female anatomy and how the sexual act resulted in conception. She told how this ultimately led to the birth of the child. When she finished after about fifteen minutes, she breathed a sigh of relief and expectantly waited for her child's reaction. The child responded, "But Mommy, I didn't want to know all that. I just wanted to know what hospital I was born in!"

The message in this anecdote is clear. Try to determine exactly what your child wants to know. Some children may not even know what answers they are looking for. So just start answering briefly, and then ask if that's what they wanted to know. Continue from there.

Be careful not to frighten your child. Children have great imaginations. You don't want your answers to get blown out of proportion. Telling your child you have a problem with your heart might be quite anxiety provoking. Without completely understanding the nature of the problem, your child might fear you'll have a heart attack and die. This will require much reassurance (probably like you were reassured when you were diagnosed!). But remember: You do want your child to continue to talk to you about your condition. If you show that you accept MVP (as much as you can) and the way it affects you, and that you even welcome questions about it, this will greatly benefit your relationship with your child.

"Will You Die?"

This is an inevitable question. Whenever a child knows that a parent has a serious medical problem, he or she may worry. It may be frightening for your child to see you having more difficulty functioning. You'll have to handle this very carefully. Children become petrified thinking about the death of a parent. They don't understand what you're going through and they will certainly be afraid. Reassure them that you're not going to die. Even if you don't always believe this 100 percent yourself, this is what they need to hear.

Remember, in general, people don't die because of mitral valve prolapse. But what if it is hard for you to tell your child that you will not die because you're not convinced yourself? (Children are very perceptive; they'll recognize your fears.) It might be a good idea, therefore, to speak to a professional (your physician or your child's pediatrician, for example) and include him or her in the discussion.

Spending Time

One of the hardest parts of coping with children is handling their disappointment when you can't do all that they'd like you to do. You want to be a good parent. But what does that entail? Most parents believe that they must spend lots of time with their children, taking them places and doing things with them. If this doesn't happen, parents may feel guilty. But mitral valve prolapse can be restrictive. The fatigue, especially, may prevent you from doing a lot of what you'd like to do.

How do you solve this dilemma? How do you explain to your child that you can't take him or her somewhere, or that you can't do what you had promised? (Children don't want to understand when they're upset.) Making deals can help. Explain to your children that you're not able to do as much as you'd like to. Come to an agreement with them about some enjoyable activity you can do together when you're feeling better. This arrangement will show your children that you're aware of their unhappiness and want to help.

Try to spend "quality" time with your children—special time when you really share feelings and activities. You shouldn't be as concerned about "quantity" time—the number of minutes or hours you spend with them. If your time together is precious, then this is much more important than the amount of time. Your children will do just fine. Talking with your children and being open with them is another important factor in helping them to handle your medical condition.

COPING WITH ADOLESCENTS

Coping with adolescents can be very different from coping with children. Because adolescents are older and can read more complex material, they can therefore read most of what has been written for adults. They can ask questions if anything they read is too complicated. However, the main difficulty in coping with adolescents is recognizing their unique needs.

The Declaration of Independence

This is the age at which teenagers begin to assert their independence. Look out, world! The future generation is coming! Adolescents want to start moving away from the family setting and its responsibilities. Under normal circumstances, this can create problems in many homes. Your MVP can cause even more problems. Why? Because of this, your adolescent may have to help out more than usual with daily routines and chores. At the same time, the adolescent wants to do less and be away more. What a bummer!

For example, fifteen-year-old Douglas feels guilty about not helping out more at home, but feels that giving in is a sign of weakness (heaven forbid!). This causes Douglas a lot of anguish, which, of course, he doesn't want to discuss with his parents. The need to escape seems even greater. So, dear parent, imagine how helpful it can be for you to be aware of your adolescent's feelings. Take the initiative and offer a reasonable compromise. Just showing that you understand will help. Maybe things won't seem so hopeless to the adolescent, after all.

The Need for Friends

Adolescents are usually less interested in spending time with family members, and more interested in being with friends. That should make it easier, but it may still be difficult for an adolescent to deal with a parent's MVP. Even if the adolescent's friends don't know about your condition, the adolescent may be much more sensitive to the situation. Does this sound strange? Most adolescents want to impress their friends. Somehow, having a parent who has a medical problem doesn't quite "fit the bill." Of course, there are some adolescents who are more mature and open about it. The extent of their love for their parent and a sound family relationship minimize the problem. They may sometimes end relationships with those friends who cannot understand the situation. Unfortunately, however, this is not often the case.

Another problem for your adolescent is transportation (that means you!). Many adolescents count on their parents to drive them to friends' houses, parties, meetings, and so on. But you may not be available (or able) to chauffeur your teenager around as much. As a result, you may feel guilty and believe you're not being a good parent. Your teenager, thinking less of you and more of himself or herself, can become upset or even angry. Your teenager also may feel guilty, either because of recognizing this selfishness, or because of feeling like too much of a burden. The best thing to do is to talk it out.

Talking to Your Adolescent

Understanding the needs of your adolescent can open the doors to much better communication. However, if you want your talking to be helpful, treat the adolescent like an adult. This will provide the best response. Think about the concerns of your adolescent regarding your condition. Reassuring him or her may help. If your adolescent feels comfortable talking to you about your MVP, encourage it. But remember to respect the rights of those adolescents who would rather not discuss it.

Finally . . .

Your adolescent may shoulder more responsibilities, but this may cause more problems. Some adolescents will be able to deal effectively with their burdens, but some won't. They may simply be unable to handle the pressure. If your adolescent must take on any additional adult responsibilities or jobs because of your condition, consider that he or she may also be ready to enjoy some more adult privileges and pleasures. How can you require teenagers to fulfill adult responsibilities and then restrict them to teenage privileges? If you're apprehensive about their maturity, keep in mind that if they're old enough to do adult chores, they might enjoy some adult privileges as well (within reason, of course). Adolescents will usually be more willing to help out if they know that they will be treated and trusted in a more grown-up way.

COPING WITH PARENTS

Parents have a very hard time dealing with mitral valve prolapse, or any medical illness or condition, in their child (even in an adult "child"). This makes coping harder for you, too. Why? You don't want your parents to suffer or be upset. You'd probably feel guilty about their suffering.

If your relationship with your parents is good, then you're among the lucky ones. But what if you normally have difficulty dealing with your parents? Having MVP doesn't help! Regardless of the type of relationship you've had, how have your parents treated you since your diagnosis? Do they ignore or minimize your condition? Or do they smother you?

The Ignorers

Patty, a twenty-one-year-old secretary living with her parents, was diagnosed with MVP two years ago. Since her diagnosis, her parents have been showing less and less concern about her condition When Patty says that she has some pain, her mother just tells her to "take her pills." When tired, her father tells her that "staying in bed won't accomplish anything." If looks could kill. . . .

Besides all of this, they don't ask questions. Even worse, they don't show any interest when she wants to tell them something about it.

Parents who ignore or play down your medical condition often do this because they can't deal with it. They can't face the fact that their child is sick. They can't accept the possibility that it might have something to do with them. How? They may be afraid that they did something to contribute to the illness or condition. Or maybe they think you inherited the illness or condition from them. (After all, MVP can run in families . . . !)

Even if these thoughts are untrue, it doesn't eliminate the worry underlying such thoughts. To avoid these unpleasant feelings, they may try to deny your having mitral valve prolapse. They might minimize it, hoping it will all go away.

The Smotherers

Since Diana was told she had MVP, her mother has visited her on an average of four times per week. This would be nice, except: 1. Her mother lives forty-five minutes away by car. 2. Her mother has emphysema and needs her rest. 3. Diana doesn't want to see her so often. You see, Diana is thirty-one, hasn't lived at home for thirteen years, and often disagrees with her mother's opinions (especially regarding what activities she should participate in and how much rest she should get). Diana certainly feels smothered.

Parents who smother believe that if you have any kind of problem, they must take care of you. Having mitral valve prolapse certainly fits this requirement. It doesn't matter what your marital status is or how old you are. What matters to them is that they are your parents. They are responsible for you and must take care of you. The fact that you can take care of yourself doesn't matter. They'll call frequently, asking how you're doing. They'll want to know what they can do to help. They may come over as often as possible to make sure you're okay.

Whether they come or not, they'll constantly bombard you with questions about your health and activities. What can you do, short of moving out of town and taking on a new identity?

Remember what we said before? It really helps to see a situation through someone else's eyes! Don't you think this holds true here, too? Look at yourself and your condition through the eyes of your parents. How do you think they feel? They care about you. What do they see? They see their child, needing them! You don't have to agree with them, but understanding this will help you talk to them. Looking at your condition through their eyes also will help any discussions you may have with them as you try to explain how you feel. It's fine to let them know that it bothers you when they do certain things. You'll feel great if your discussions are more productive.

What if Talking Doesn't Help?

If you have tried to talk to your parents and haven't succeeded, at least you've tried. That will help you feel a little better! At least you won't feel like you should do more to convince them to switch to your way of thinking! What do you do then? Concentrate more on helping yourself feel better, regardless of whether they understand or not. If they're unhappy with you because you seem to be rejecting their well-meant intentions, so be it.

By the way, if you're unhappy with parents who are ignorers, you'd probably love them to smother you for awhile. And, if you don't like smothering parents, the thought of being left alone is probably very exciting. There's rarely a perfect solution. No one gets along with everyone all the time. Instead of complaining about your parents' faults, try to look at the positives in their behavior. You'll feel better about doing this, too.

How Much Should You Tell Your Parents?

You know your parents. You know how they react to things. What would you really like to share with them? Would you like to tell them how you're feeling at a particular time? You probably know how they'll react to good news and bad news, and how they deal with unpleasantness. How will you handle their reactions? All these factors will help you to decide how much to tell them.

Sometimes, it's easier to talk with one parent rather than the other. You might tell one parent what's bothering you, and let that parent tell the other. For example, your mother may be able to get through to your father better than you can. This will help everybody.

You might wish you could share unpleasant feelings with a parent because of the reassurance it would bring. It's nice to know that you don't have to face something unpleasant alone. However, what if your parents can't readily accept your problems even if they might want to? It may be more detrimental for you to tell them things that they can't handle. So don't impulsively tell them anything. Think and analyze. Try to understand what you want to share and what their reactions may be. It's worth the effort. By spending a little time to figure out what's best, you can help yourself feel a lot better. You'll probably improve your relationship with your parents, as well.

25

Friends and Colleagues

Aside from family, the most important people you'll have to deal with are friends and colleagues. Are there any suggestions for coping with these important people? Of course!

COPING WITH YOUR FRIENDS

What reactions have your friends had about your mitral valve prolapse? How many of them even know that you have it? Of those, how many really know what MVP is all about? They may have read about it, and at first, they may have thought they understood MVP. But because they weren't physically affected, they might not have been able to really understand what you were experiencing. Some wanted to learn more; some wanted to forget what little they knew.

Some friends may be very supportive (maybe too supportive!). Other friends may not be supportive enough, something that can bother you even more. Your own mood may determine their reactions.

If you don't want friends around, if you don't want them close to you, or if you don't want them asking questions, let them know this. They probably will respect your wishes. But perhaps they won't be there when you really do want them around. It's important for you to strike a balance. You may simply want to explain that your feelings change and to ask that they please bear with you. You hope they'll understand the fluctuation of your feelings.

Apprehension Keeps Them Away

Friends may not know what to say to you. What should they ask you? How should they talk to you? This can cause so much tension that they don't even want to be with you. They may be so uneasy that they feel, "Why bother?"

Friends may be afraid to call because they don't know how you're feeling. They don't want to run the risk of stirring up unpleasant feelings for you (or for themselves, if they don't know how to respond). On the other hand, there may be times when friends keep asking you how you're feeling and you'd really like to be left alone. Many friendships are lost or hurt because of misunderstandings. These misunderstandings usually involve uncertainty on the part of you or your friends in approaching each other.

Showing Concern

Can anything be done, or are you going to be a hermit for the rest of your life? Don't despair. There are things you can do to improve the situation. Try to establish ground rules with your friends. Tell them how you feel. If you are the kind of person who likes to be asked how you feel, let your friends know. If you'd rather not be asked, let your friends know that, too. If your feelings fluctuate (sometimes feeling talkative about your condition, but at other times feeling reluctant even to think about it), let your friends know. Your changing feelings may be harder for friends to deal with, so let them know that they should talk to you the way they really want to. You'll let them know if and when you're having trouble.

Clear up the question marks. If you tell your friends how you feel and what your needs and desires are, fewer unknowns will exist. The uneasiness about what to do or say, which can hurt friendships, will be reduced. Your friends will become more aware of your needs and will feel closer to you and less afraid.

Changing Plans

Don't you love having to change plans with a friend at the last minute because you're so tired that you can't even move? Probably not. So you can understand how your friends might feel if this has to happen.

This doesn't have to be so. Good friends, who understand or at least try to understand what you're going through, probably will be able to accept these changes. Others may be less willing to put up with them.

Kathy hated when she and her husband made plans with friends and she had to bow out because of symptoms of mitral valve prolapse. What made it worse was that her husband went ahead with the plans anyway! She had to stay home alone because no one else wanted to change their plans. So not only was there friction between Kathy and her friends, but more marital arguments were resulting as well. Since this may be an unfortunate part of living with MVP, you'll have to hope that discussing these problems with your friends will result in increased tolerance and understanding that will maintain some good friendships.

Asking for Help

As you learn to live with MVP, do you feel a greater need to call on your friends for help? What if there are times when you need help cleaning the house, getting places, taking care of children, purchasing groceries, or doing other things? Are you becoming more selfish? No, but it may seem that way to you. Of course, selfishness is not the reason. After all, if you ask for help more often, it's because you're less able to do things independently. You'd probably like to be able to do these things yourself, but it just may not be possible. The reality is: There are certain things you must take care of. If you don't do them, then what? So if you need help, reach out for it. That's better than pushing yourself too much and suffering the consequences.

If your friends complain or show resentment, try to talk it over with them. Don't wait until a friendship is destroyed to realize that built-up problems should have been discussed earlier, when the conflict could have been resolved. If you try and nothing helps, remember this: If your friends still don't understand, what kind of friends are they, anyway?

Asking for Help Appropriately!

If you do need help, figure out who to ask and what they should do. If your friend Myrna loves children, it probably would be better to ask her for help with the kids. If you know that Maureen suffers from "supermarketitis," requiring daily therapeutic visits to the local food emporium, then asking her to go for groceries shouldn't bother her at all. If Mario has a driving phobia, don't ask him to chauffeur you around! Try to arrange for a proper fit when asking for help.

Older, longer-lasting friendships also tend to be stronger and more resilient. Such friends probably will be more receptive if you ask for favors. Newer or more casual friend probably should not be burdened as much. Without giving a friendship a chance to become firmly planted on your hook, you may lose your prize fish—a good, long-lasting friendship. Don't come on too strong. You might think, "But can't they see that I need help?" The answer is, "Not necessarily."

Don't feel like you must do everything yourself. There's nothing wrong with reaching out for help.

But you'll feel better if you try to evaluate who to ask for what kind of help. (By the way, when you feel up to it, a nice way to show your appreciation is through an unsolicited gift or gesture.)

Losing Friends

What if it just doesn't work out the way you want? People you thought were your friends don't call or visit. Some are "turned off" by your having a medical problem. Maybe they just can't deal with it. Others seem reluctant to make any plans with you, saying, "Let's wait and see how you feel." It's sad, but in some cases it just can't be avoided. It's not your decision! And you don't want it to be your problem!

Why might this have happened? Was your friend uncomfortable about being with you? Was your friend unsure of what to say or do? Was your friend unable to handle any changes of plans? Whatever the reason, you've probably learned a hard, unpleasant lesson. Although you may feel sad, you can't change someone else's feelings. Be reassured that most people who lose friends do make new ones. You really don't want a "friend" who is uncomfortable with you.

If a friend or lover cannot handle your condition, you may feel like you've been rejected. This can be devastating! You may feel that not only have you been rejected, but that you will not be able to develop any other meaningful relationships. This is not true. You are still the same person you were before, except for the ways that your condition has affected you physically. Keep telling yourself that so you can restore any confidence that may have been shaken by this unfortunate rejection.

Usually, however, if rejection occurs or if a relationship breaks up, it couldn't have been too strong to begin with. Many weak relationships have broken up because of medical problems. A sturdy relationship, even if it has to go through some rough times, probably will end up even stronger than before. Remember, you want a friend who likes you the way you are, mitral valve prolapse and all! And there are plenty of wonderful, understanding people out there. So don't give up!

COPING WITH COLLEAGUES

We've discussed some of the work-related problems you may have if you have mitral valve prolapse. If you know you're going to work, what kinds of problems might you encounter? You're going to spend several hours each day in contact with the people you work with. You'll certainly want to feel comfortable around them. Let's discuss some ways in which you might encounter difficulties in getting along with your colleagues.

Being There!

If you have to curtail your working hours, or if you find that you are absent from work more frequently because of MVP, you may encounter some bitterness or resentment. Tammy was a thirty-eight-year old executive secretary who had worked in the same office for ten years. Because of some of the symptoms of mitral valve prolapse, she found it necessary to reduce her eight-hour-a-day work schedule to four hours. This plan was endorsed by her supervisors, but was not accepted graciously by her colleagues. Many of them would have preferred working on a similar kind of part-time basis! This caused bitterness and strain in her working relationships. Some people just don't want to understand what's happening to you and why. They may feel that you're taking advantage of the situation. Hopefully this won't happen.

What about the attitudes of your colleagues? Hopefully, if you are comfortable with yourself, others will be, too. Many colleagues will take your condition in stride, and won't even think about it. This assumes, of course, that these people know about your condition.

But what if you don't want to tell anyone? Unless nosy colleagues ask questions, you may decide not to even bother telling them. Obviously, there is no requirement that you do so. And they won't see much evidence of MVP, unless they have X-ray vision!

Would it help to provide your colleagues with some basic information on mitral valve prolapse? It might, although it may not necessarily improve their attitude toward you or your condition. In addition, reading about something doesn't always lead to understanding. However, at least you'll feel better knowing that you've tried to help them understand more about MVP. If they don't, they don't. Remember: You can't change somebody else. If a colleague (or anybody else, for that matter) can't handle or understand what's going on, that's his or her problem. You can try to educate people about MVP, but don't make it your problem. If you've got an employer with an open mind, that's terrific. Don't be as concerned about other people who don't understand what you're going through. Concentrate more on doing the best you can.

Cooperative Colleague Compromises

Elaine found it impossible to complete all of her required work. She was afraid she'd lose her job. However, rather than giving up, she was able to make an arrangement with one of her colleagues who was willing to assist her in completing her tasks whenever she felt physically unable to do so alone. As a result, much of the pressure on Elaine's shoulders was removed.

Occasionally, you may find that you are unable to complete all of your work. Try to work out some kind of an arrangement with a colleague. This may sound strange (even uncomfortable) at first, but it can result in even better relationships and understanding among your colleagues. You have nothing to lose. The worst they could say is, "No! I won't help."

Whether you need to work or you enjoy working, you'll certainly want to minimize any potential occupational problems caused by your condition. Take one day at a time. Don't worry about problems that have not, and may never, occur. If your MVP does cause a problem, be precise in identifying exactly what it is so that you can employ the best strategies to resolve it.

26

Your Physician

How do you feel about your physician? (What a question!) Some people see physicians as gods. Others feel that they're rich, unconcerned, cold professionals who don't really want to help. Of course, there are other opinions. What's your feeling?

Your opinion plays a role in determining how your treatment progresses. You may find that your feelings toward your physician (or physicians in general) have changed since your diagnosis. Some people with MVP don't have as much confidence in their physicians, probably because they haven't been cured yet!

Many individuals question what type of doctor they should be working with if they have been diagnosed with MVP. Some people feel that a cardiologist would be the most appropriate type of physician, since a cardiologist specializes in heart disease and is most familiar with MVP and its symptoms. This may not always be necessary. It may depend on the severity of the symptoms and your preference for who treats you, among other factors. Internists and general practitioners may certainly be able to help you if the condition is affecting you in a way that doesn't require a specialist. In this case, the more important considerations in determining what doctor you'll be seeing would be compassion and the willingness to work with you.

THE IMPORTANCE OF DOCTOR-PATIENT RELATIONSHIPS

Regardless of your opinions of the medical profession, it is realistically impossible to stay away from your physician if you have MVP. Instead, you'll want a good working relationship. You have to see your physician more often than someone who does not have a chronic medical problem. Because of the symptoms that you may experience because of mitral valve prolapse, you'll certainly benefit from trying to develop the best possible relationship with your physician. That takes awareness, understanding, and effort on your part.

You need a good relationship with your physician for a number of reasons. Your physician will help to manage your MVP symptoms, to decrease the risk of complications, and to give you guidelines for any changes in lifestyle that are beneficial (or necessary).

PROBLEMS WITH THE DOCTOR-PATIENT RELATIONSHIP

Many physicians are much more comfortable in treating patients when symptoms of a medical problem are noticeable, tangible, and observable. With MVP, other than the anatomical structural problems of the mitral valve, there may be many symptoms, such as anxiety, palpitations, or chest pain, that just aren't as observable as one might want them to be.

Why might many individuals with MVP have a difficult time dealing with physicians? Many people spend a lot of time trying to find out what is wrong with them. Many people with MVP have seen a number of physicians before they are ultimately diagnosed. Many individuals complain that the symptoms that they do report receive very little attention or even credibility.

Much of what doctors know about MVP leads them to believe that it is, for the most part, a comparatively benign problem. Therefore, if you present them with a diagnosis of MVP, they may tell you that it is nothing to worry about. It may be especially difficult if you're experiencing symptoms of MVP, but MVP has not yet been diagnosed. It's not too pleasant if, in these cases, the physicians feel that the symptoms are more in your head!

But there is another problem. Virtually any person who is told that there is a problem with his or her heart (even if it's MVP) will experience some anxiety. Virtually any person with MVP who experiences chest pain will worry about whether or not this is MVP or something that is more serious and requires attention. There also may be some anxiety that is related to the imbalance (even if it is minor) in the autonomic nervous system, a problem that is often associated with MVP. Physicians must be sensitive to these concerns and not be so fast to dismiss what is being experienced.

Wouldn't you prefer to deal with a physician who will take the time to carefully explain what MVP is all about, to tell you why you may experience discomfort, and to answer other questions? Wouldn't you also like to be reassured that MVP need not be serious? On the other hand, you're probably not thrilled if the physician simply says, "Oh, you have MVP, don't worry about it—everything will be okay." And then you walk out, worrying that there is something wrong with your heart, and wondering about what might happen next.

It may seem that physicians don't know best, and that you, more than anyone else, know how you feel. Because of all these feelings, not to mention the rising costs of medical care, physicians frequently bear the brunt of much hostility. But physicians do want to help. They probably feel as frustrated as you do when they don't know what to suggest. It's unpleasant for anyone to admit that the answers are out of reach, especially when that person knows you are relying on them.

Are you hesitant about speaking to your physician? Perhaps you're afraid of being put in the hospital if your physician finds out how you've been feeling. You might be concerned that your physician will not like the way you're taking care of yourself. You might be afraid your doctor will consider you a complainer who's "crying wolf" and may not listen if an emergency occurs. You might be apprehensive that your physician will increase your medication. Or you may be afraid that your physician won't believe what you're saying, thinking that the symptoms you are reporting are "all in your head!" Despite these concerns, you do want your physician to do the best for you. So try to be completely open and honest about the way you're feeling and what you're doing.

Want to get easily frustrated? Try calling your physician for whatever reason (whether it's an emergency or not), only to wait long hours for your call to be returned. This may be one of your criteria when searching for a physician. Make sure you feel confident in your physician's punctuality in returning your calls.

IMPROVING THE DOCTOR-PATIENT RELATIONSHIP

There are a number of ways that you can develop a better relationship with your physician. It's very important to have a certain degree of understanding for the position the physician is in. Make sure you properly communicate the way you feel. If the physician prescribes medication, for example, be patient with it. Don't expect medication to bring about instantaneous results. Sometimes it can take weeks before medication builds to the level necessary in the blood to bring about the change.

It is very important for you to demonstrate to the physician that you are actively involved in your own self-care. Don't do this in a way that creates antagonism, but rather, do so in a way that shows the physician that are interested in helping yourself. Not only will you listen to the physician, but you will be putting your own effort into the process.

Make the most of your visits. Try to be organized any time you go for an appointment. Have a list of any questions you want to ask, and jot down notes as they are answered. Discuss when it's a good idea to call if you have concerns or questions, and when it's a good idea not to. Doctors are usually cooperative, believing that this makes the office visit more efficient and time-effective.

Follow the doctor's prescribed treatment program. If there are things that you're not sure of or you're uncomfortable with, question the doctor about those things. But when you come to an agreement on the treatment program, by all means follow it. Any problems that occur as a result of your treatment program should be reported to your physician so changes can take place.

People like to believe that their physicians know what they're talking about. This doesn't mean, however, that you must blindly accept everything that's said. For the most part, physicians respect the patient who asks questions. Disagreement doesn't mean that your physician will throw you out, or even back down. But if you are unsure of why something is being suggested, question it. It's very important to be honest with your physician (as well as with yourself!). If you don't like a particular medication, or if it does not seem to be working for you, speak up. Don't hold back. You do have the right to question. In fact, you have the obligation to question. Being unsure is a certain way to be tense. And relaxation is very important.

After you've lived with MVP for a while, you'll better learn when you should call and when it's not as necessary. Certain symptoms, such as intense chest pain, may require you to immediately contact your physician. Other symptoms, such as mild shortness of breath, may not have to be reported immediately. Discuss this with your physician. Find out his or her feelings about your calling if you have problems. Ask about the kind of things that should be phoned in. Also ask when the best time is to call.

GETTING SECOND OPINIONS

Because you may not absolutely agree with everything your physician says, and because no physician knows all, you might want a second opinion. There should be a justifiable reason for this. But many people are worried about hurting their physician's feelings. Don't look at it that way. Think logically. Most physicians will accept your desire to get a second opinion. It will either confirm what they believe, or will point out the need for further discussion.

If your physician objects to your getting a second opinion, you should certainly question why. This does not suggest, however, that you should make it a habit of going for second opinions. Nor should you continually shop around for the "ideal" physician. No such person exists.

Remember that there is a difference between changing physicians and seeking a second opinion. A second opinion is something that is done to validate the treatments prescribed by the previous doctor. It's also done to determine whether or not a relatively extreme suggestion for a treatment or procedure would be beneficial in a given case.

YOU'RE NOT "LOCKED IN"

Some people have a lot of trouble with the idea of changing physicians; others seem to change physicians more than socks! If you are considering changing, ask yourself why. Are you changing because the doctor does not give you the appropriate information or the appropriate time? Are you changing because the doctor seems to be hostile? In any case, regardless of your answer to this question, be sure to ask yourself if there is anything that you may have said or done that contributed to your doctor's hostility. This should be carefully considered before continuing with your decision to change.

In addition, before changing doctors, consider whether or not the relationship can be salvaged. Many people find that if they sit down and talk to the doctor about their concerns in a constructive, positive way, problems can be ironed out, and changing doctors is no longer necessary.

Don't try to accomplish this over the telephone or at the tail end of a regular examination. Set up a separate consultation appointment where you can sit down and discuss things that you are concerned about. Many people may be unable to do this, however. They may feel that they're not comfortable saying something negative to their physician.

If you're not happy with your physician, you're not under any obligation to continue seeing him or her. Don't continue a relationship unless it's a good one. Don't continue going to a particular physician if you feel you can't ask questions, if you feel intimidated, or if you feel you can't call if there is a problem. Don't stick with your physician if you don't have confidence in what you're told, whether it's about treatment or medication. Finally, don't continue seeing your physician if you feel that he or she doesn't care about you and does not have your best interests at heart.

Your honesty is part of a good professional relationship. If your questions or disagreements hurt the relationship, or if you are afraid of being honest, then this relationship may not be the one for you.

You may want to discuss all of this with your doctor before making any moves. This might straighten things out and improve the relationship. But if it doesn't, remember that you're looking out for your health. You want the support of a physician who can meet most of your needs.

There are actually three options if you're not happy with your physician. Option number one is to continue to stay and be miserable with the doctor under the present circumstances. Option number two is to learn how to be more assertive so that you can constructively say the things you want to say. And option number three is to simply change doctors without trying to do anything to salvage the existing relationship. Only you can decide how to proceed.

27

Comments From Others

As Ralph Kramden of *The Honeymooners* would say, "Some people have a *B-I-G MOUTH!*" You may agree with this when you think of some of the comments you hear from people around you. They may know you have a medical problem, but that doesn't mean they know how to talk to you about it, or what to say. They may say things that they feel are right, witty, intelligent, or even sympathetic. But you may think otherwise! There are times when a certain comment might make you want to implant your knuckles in the speaker's teeth! Or a comment might make you wonder if you're talking to a graduate of the Ignoramus School of Tactlessness.

But why are you reading all this? As you know by now, you cannot change other people. You cannot correct their lack of sensitivity or improve the way they talk. What you can do is learn how to cope with some of the ridiculous comments that you may hear.

ARE OTHERS BEING CRUEL?

Most people really say things out of sincere concern. They may be trying to make you feel better, show their support, or show an interest in you by questioning how you're feeling. Does that mean you must always be receptive to their questions and respond to all of them seriously? It would be nice. The problem is that hearing the same questions over and over can begin to get on your nerves. Initially, you may try to gently respond to comments or questions, or politely change the subject. However, this does not always work. Some people avoid this by simply not telling anyone about their condition.

For the purpose of this chapter, let's assume that we're discussing those comments that you can't avoid from people who haven't yet learned to tune into your feelings. If you haven't experienced this, that's great! But read on anyway. You never know when what you read might come in handy!

HOW TO RESPOND

Many of the things that people say to you may be legitimate comments, but may bug you just the same. Others may not even deserve proper answers. Still others may be said without considering your feelings. But it doesn't matter why the comment is inappropriate. What really matters is how you handle these comments so that you feel comfortable. There are three ways this can be done.

The first way is to ignore the comments. This is not always easy, especially if the person is waiting for your response or seems genuinely insulted by your lack of response. How do you get him or her to stop asking (besides buying a muzzle!)? Change the subject or walk away—ignore the question.

The second way is to try to answer in a rational and intelligent way, explaining your answer, how you feel, or what you sincerely want to communicate to the other person. But now you may feel like you're banging your head against a wall. What if you just can't convince the other person of what you're trying to say? Such frustration can be painful! There's a limit as to how many times you can try to explain something clearly, and not have it understood or accepted, before you explode. (And this isn't good for your physical health, either!)

What if the first two ways don't do the trick? There's got to be a better way, and there is. The third way is to respond humorously. What does this mean? If someone says something unreasonable to you or asks you a foolish question that can't really be answered logically, you'll accomplish very little by ignoring it or trying to reasonably explain your feelings. You don't know if your answer will be accepted or if the interrogation will continue. So, in many cases, the third option may be best. This is called "paradoxical intention." The idea behind it is that the person is asking or saying something that is really unanswerable. So you're going to have a little fun with your response. Let's see how it works.

Handling the "Big Mouth" Syndrome

What might you hear? And how should you handle it? Remember, the best response is one that will educate the "commenter." You'd like to explain your situation nicely, in a non-offensive, sincere way. But you're only human. So how can you respond when you get fed up? Read on . . .

"But You Look So Good . . ."

You've awakened in the morning after a full night's sleep, but you still feel tired. You have a lot to do to get ready for your day's activities, but you don't feel like doing much of anything. Your husband walks into the room and asks you if you are ready to get up. You tell him that you're not ready yet; you'd like to rest some more because you feel really lousy. He looks at you and says, "How can you feel lousy? You look so good."

Wouldn't it be nice if you had enough energy at this point to pop him in the nose? Any time that your fatigue makes you feel like your muscles have been drained of energy, it can be very frustrating to be told that you should do more because you look good. This is one of those statements that's hard to ignore, but it's just as hard and impractical to try to answer it rationally. So how can you respond to this statement humorously? You might say, "Yes, I know I look good. You can call my plastic surgeon and thank him." Or you can say, "Yes, I look good. Wait until you see me without my mask on." Notice that in both of these cases, you're agreeing with the person first, and then you're saying something humorous. Isn't that better than saying, "How can you say I look good when I feel so awful?"

"You Look Awful!"

On the other side of the coin, it can be just as upsetting when somebody says, "Wow, you look lousy!" You may feel lousy but you certainly don't want to be reminded of it. You surely don't want to think that the way you feel is so obvious to others. You'd like to at least believe that you look okay to those around you. Even if it's said sympathetically, being told that you don't look well may be insulting. So what do you say? You might respond, "Thank you, so do you!" Or, "Yes, I know. I've worked hard to look that way." Or if you're really in a cynical mood, you might say, "I know I look lousy. That comes from hearing people tell me this!" Of course, you could always say, "That makes sense, since I don't feel so hot, either!"

"You Think Too Much!"

You are quietly sitting in a chair trying to regain some energy because you really feel exhausted. Somebody comes over to you and asks what's wrong. You try to explain that you're feeling very tired and you're trying to gather some energy. In a concerned way, the person says, "You're spending too much time thinking about yourself. Just get up and do something. Soon you won't even remember that you're not feeling well!" How do you react to that? Do you jump out of your chair? Of course not. If you had the energy to get out of your chair, would you have been slumped there in the first place? Do you sit there and try to explain that you're feeling lousy? No, because you probably won't be believed. So how do you respond humorously? You might say, "I would like to get up, but somebody put fast-drying glue on the chair, and I'm stuck forever!" Or you might respond, "I'm trying to set a Guinness World Record for the most time I can spend in this chair." Or you might say, "Do you know how much energy it takes to remain in this chair, when what I really want to do is to get up and knock your block off?" Obviously, the type of response you use depends on how angry or irritated you feel.

Remember: For this approach to work best, you want to respond in a lighthearted way. This will show the person making the comment that you're fine, but you just don't appreciate what he or she is saying.

"You Go to Too Many Doctors!"

Let's say a friend finds out that you have still another doctor's appointment. You may hear, "You're just going to too many doctors.

Why don't you stop going all over the place and just do what you have to do." How do you respond to this? You might respond by saying, "Yes, and I'll keep going to different doctors until I exhaust my bank account." Or you might say, "I like to go to a lot of doctors. The smell of the antiseptic waiting room excites me!" Or, "Do you realize how many of their children I'm putting through college this way?"

"What's the Matter With Your Heart?"

Some people really don't understand what MVP is all about. (Really!) All they understand is that you've got some kind of problem with your heart. So, of course, they ask about it. This kind of comment usually does show genuine concern. Under some circumstances you might want to simply explain that your heart itself is fine, but one of the valves is not working properly and you're experiencing some of the symptoms that can result from this. But if this is the twenty-fourth time you've heard the same question, it's hard to respond calmly. What could you say that would not be cruel, but would still allow you to feel better about the way you handled the situation? How about, "This isn't *my* heart. It's one I borrowed from a neighbor!" Or you could say, "I don't have a heart. I gave it to the Salvation Army in July!" Or how about, "Nothing's wrong with my heart. But I'm concerned about the hearts of people who keep asking me what's wrong with mine!" This does not suggest that you be unfeeling in your answers. However, if you need to let the "commenter" know that you don't appreciate these questions, that'll do it!

"Aren't You Frightened That You'll Get a Heart Attack?"

In response to this profoundly sympathetic expression of curiosity, you might want to say, "Sure, aren't you?" Or you might want to point out that MVP pain is not the same as heart attack pain by saying, "MVP pain I can stand, because I know it's not the same as heart attack pain. But what I can't stand is the pain I get from hearing questions like these!" People will get the message. You may not like the symptoms of MVP, but at least you're learning to cope with the situation.

"What Is Mitral Valve Prolapse?"

How do you respond if somebody sarcastically says, "I never heard of mitral valve prolapse. What's that?" You might say, "Let's forget you even brought it up. Then you can keep your streak going!" Or you could say, "I never heard of it either. How's the weather?" Don't forget: You really don't want to hurt the person's feelings by being sarcastic. However, coping with comments from others can be one of the hardest things about living with MVP. There are times when being gentle and tactful with others is less important than helping yourself handle comments without becoming aggravated.

If the person asks why you sound sarcastic, you can explain that you're not trying to be that way, but that the comment or question you just heard was so ridiculous that you figured the person was trying to be funny. So you decided to have some fun, too! But if the person really wants to know how you feel . . .

You won't always have to use this technique, but you may want to be prepared anyway. You'll always come across someone who will say or ask something ridiculous. However, as you learn to feel better about your responses to comments, you'll find that you can handle them more calmly. You won't have to use sarcastic responses, and you'll have more fun with humorous, enjoyable ones. And maybe you'll keep more people on your "friend" list, rather than on your "you know what" list.

What if you're thinking, "I could never say those things. It's just not my style." Well, you don't always have to. But you can at least *think* these comments. Even that will help you to feel better!

OTHER LOVABLE COMMENTS

What are some of the other comments that you may hear? How many of these have come your way? "Is mitral valve prolapse fatal?"; "Why don't you quit your job?"; "You should exercise more!"; Are you sure you can walk up those stairs?"; "Rest. Don't do anything."; "What did the doctor say?"; "Why do you keep holding your chest?"; "What is the prognosis?"; "Wow, have you changed!"; "You must miss the way it was."; "What's the matter with you?"; "Can I help you?"; "I certainly don't envy you."; "If you would eat right, you'd feel better!"; "Why don't you try my doctor?"; "Your having mitral valve prolapse is the worst thing I ever heard!"

IS THAT ALL?

It would fill volumes to include all of the comments that you might hear from well-meaning friends or relatives. By reading these examples, you can at least get an idea of how to respond in a humorous way. Look over this list. Can you come up with some additional goodies? You don't want to be cynical or cruel. Rather, you want to show the speaker that you're feeling well enough to respond light-heartedly.

A FINAL COMMENT

One of the most common and yet most irritating comments that you may hear has been saved for last. Imagine somebody who is supposedly sympathetic and trying to help you feel better, turning to you with eyes full of compassion and concern, saying, "I heard of someone who died from mitral valve prolapse!" As you turn to walk away, you respond, "I heard of someone who died for telling someone with mitral valve prolapse what you just told me!" You walk away, head held high and a smile on your face, leaving the astonished well-wisher behind you.

28

Sex and
Mitral Valve Prolapse

This chapter is not rated R for Restricted. Rather, it is rated E for Essential. Why? If you are sexually active, you certainly don't want mitral valve prolapse to have an impact on your sex life.

Has MVP decreased your sexual appetite or ability? Many people with mitral valve prolapse experience a decreased interest in sex. This doesn't necessarily mean there's something wrong with them. As a matter of fact, decreased sexual interest is common for many people with chronic medical problems.

Any change in sexual desire can have an important bearing on the closeness of the relationship with your partner. What kind of sexual relationship did you have before you were diagnosed? (I'm not being nosy. You don't have to write and tell me!) Was it a solid one, or was it on shaky ground? If you had a good sexual relationship, you'll have an easier time getting over any obstacles that MVP may have thrown into your sex life. If your sexual relationship wasn't good, it is unlikely that having mitral valve prolapse will make it better! You may need some professional help to keep things from breaking down altogether. But all hope is not lost. If you unite with your partner to work things out together, reassuring each other, relearning how to please each other, and showing a desire for each other, progress can certainly be made.

WHERE'S THE PROBLEM?

Let's talk about what the problems might be. There can be both physiological and psychological reasons for changes in your sexual appetite. Physiological problems are better suited to specific treatments. Psychological problems are harder to deal with (ah, there's the rub). Let's explore some of the different possibilities.

Physical Problems

Can physical problems alter your interest in sex? Yes, depending on the kind of person you are, and the degree to which MVP is affecting you.

For some people with MVP, especially if they're experiencing symptoms of MVP syndrome, sex may be affected. Why? The autonomic nervous system plays an important role in two of the most important components of sexual activity, namely arousal and orgasm. Any imbalance in the autonomic nervous system may cause difficulties in either or both of these components. But remember, not everybody with the condition will experience all MVP symptoms.

What other factors in MVP can cause problems with sex? Several symptoms of mitral valve prolapse may get in the way.

Fatigue can be a factor. If you're tired, you're going to be less interested in sexual activity. This can be a real headache! (Sorry about that!) But if you're uncomfortable or fatigued, hanky-panky will just have to be put on hold. Is this a poor choice of words? Actually, it may be an excellent idea. After all, just holding each other can be wonderful, too!

If you're experiencing chest pain, you certainly may not be too sexually motivated! You may be concerned that any strenuous activity may exacerbate this pain. (It doesn't have to happen this way, but any concern you may have can surely decrease your desire.) Of course, there can be very pleasant romantic activities without undue physical strain when you're with an understanding partner.

What about drugs? Sexual problems may be caused by such medication as painkillers, sedatives, and tranquilizers, or by other types of "drugs" like alcohol. It's true that small amounts of any of these may make you feel more relaxed (increasing the possibility of sex), but too much can work against you. The use of alcohol is notorious in reducing sexual abilities because of its effect on the body.

Some drugs can have a direct effect on sexual desire. For example, certain medications (such as tranquilizers, which reduce your anxiety) can suppress sexual desire or your ability to achieve orgasm. Antihypertensive medication may also have an effect on sexual performance.

Going Out of Your Head? (Psychological Problems)

Your body isn't the only thing that may affect your sexual interest. Your mind also comes into the picture.

What's the most important sex organ? Think hard now. The correct response is: your brain! (Did I catch you?) If a sexual problem exists that is not physiological, then it doesn't exist in your body, but in your mind.

Self-Image

Living with MVP may affect your self-esteem. Do you like yourself less because of your condition? Do you feel like you're no longer a "physically intact" human being? If you feel this way, you may be more fearful of rejection by your partner. As a result, you may reduce sexual activity simply to minimize the chances of rejection.

Because self-esteem is a necessary factor in enjoying sexual intimacy, you'll want to improve your ability to like yourself. Feeling good about yourself is very important if you want to enjoy your sexual relationships. It also will make your partner feel more comfortable. On the other hand, if you don't feel good about yourself, this also will affect your partner. This can certainly interfere with closeness!

Self-consciousness can be a big problem. How has your condition affected your perception of your sexuality? If having mitral valve prolapse makes you feel less of a person sexually (and interestingly, this is not uncommon), then you've targeted an important area to work on. Try to remember that nobody's perfect. Everybody has flaws. It makes sense to work on enhancing the way you feel about yourself.

You can try to make physical changes if this will improve your self-esteem. For example, if you are overweight, wear fashions that will trim down your appearance. If you have a big nose, apply make-up so as to give the illusion of a smaller one. Whatever the problem, there is usually a way to correct or minimize it.

But improving your mental attitude is just as important. For those problems that can't be modified, use some of the thought-changing procedures described earlier in this book. They may be the key to your future happiness!

Emotional Interference

Emotions can get in the way, too! Sexual activity may be restricted because of depression. You may be so withdrawn that you simply have no interest in sex. Anxiety concerning sex itself, the intimacy of your relationship, or performance also can hold you back. You may be afraid that you just can't "make it." You may be afraid that any sexual activity might exacerbate any MVP symptoms that you're already experiencing, or create new symptoms.

Any of these things can happen in any situation, not just with mitral valve prolapse. Fortunately, they also can be dealt with through proper awareness, interaction, improved communication, and therapy (if necessary).

Maybe you're afraid of pregnancy. If this is true, it may be hard for you to enjoy sex spontaneously. Having mitral valve prolapse can make this fear even greater. Why? You may be concerned that your child will develop mitral valve prolapse. (We'll discuss this more in the next chapter on Pregnancy.)

Pain, or more important, fear of pain, may decrease your interest in sex. For example, if you've had chest pain, it usually does go away in a while (with or without specific medical treatment). But what if you have a long memory about this pain or you're afraid that this pain may become stronger during sex? Yes, the psychological effects of the chest pain may last longer than the physiological effects.

TALK IT OVER

A very important part of sexual relationships is communication. If you and your partner can share thoughts and feelings, you'll be in much better shape to work out any sexual problems that may occur as a result of your condition. If communication problems exist, how-ever, difficulties may be very hard to resolve. It is important to discuss sexual problems with your partner. You can work through such feelings. Acknowledge any problems and discuss them with your partner. It can be very helpful to discuss these problems with your physician or other health professionals as well. In many cases, the major problem is that these feelings are kept inside and any discussion is avoided, causing your sexual life to dwindle down to nothing.

Try to maintain nice, wide-open lines of communication with your partner. Discuss any sexual problems openly. You may even want to discuss them with your physician or another professional to determine whether they are physiological or psychological. You'll then be better able to work on them.

All that has been said, of course, assumes that your interest in sex is affected by your condition, and that your partner is suffering. But what if the opposite is true? What if you still have normal sexual desires, but your partner is the one who's afraid? Maybe there's a fear of hurting you or creating additional problems. Or maybe you're regarded as a fragile flower, easily broken, and your partner is reluctant to be sexually spontaneous. This must be carefully discussed. If one-on-one attempts at working things out don't help, don't hesitate to get some professional assistance. It's well worth it.

AND NOW THE CLIMAX

Because sex is such an intimate and important part of a marriage (or any serious relationship), the whole relationship can be affected when either or both partners feel there is trouble. Try to discuss this. If necessary, include your physician in a discussion to clarify issues that may not be as readily accepted. You can still have a warm relationship even if your sex life is less active, but not if there are bitter feelings and misgivings at the same time. Understanding each other's feelings is a very important part of coping with mitral valve prolapse.

Remember: Having MVP doesn't mean that sexual activity must be reduced, curtailed, or totally eliminated! As a matter of fact, it can still be as pleasurable and important as both partners want it to be.

29

Pregnancy

To have a baby, or not to have a baby. That is the conception. Whether it is nobler (or safer) to have children may be a big question mark. Why? You may be concerned that, since MVP is genetically transmitted, your children may have a greater chance of developing the condition. You may be afraid that mitral valve prolapse will cause a difficult or unsafe pregnancy. Let's consider some of the important issues regarding pregnancy.

DOES PREGNANCY AFFECT YOUR MITRAL VALVE PROLAPSE?

Is it possible that your MVP, or your health in general, may be affected by pregnancy? After all, you reason, MVP affects your heart; what if pregnancy puts an added strain on your heart? This really isn't a problem. In fact, some people with MVP notice that symptoms of MVP may diminish or even disappear during pregnancy. This may happen because there is an increase in blood volume during pregnancy. Increased blood volume can decrease or eliminate a number of MVP symptoms.

   Unfortunately, this does not mean that any change in symptoms will be permanent (although it might be). After delivery, a reduction in blood volume may be one reason for an increase of symptoms, but symptoms may be exacerbated by the fatigue that you'll experience from long hours of taking care of your child. The best way to try to stabilize your condition both during pregnancy and after is with a proper diet and appropriate fluid intake.

DOES MITRAL VALVE PROLAPSE AFFECT YOUR PREGNANCY?

You might be concerned about whether or not pregnancy is safe if you have MVP. The reality is that there should be no effect on your pregnancy. If you have any questions, though, they should be directed toward your physician.

In all probability, the most important consideration concerns medication. You'll need to determine whether any of your medications should be discontinued. Your physician is the one who must advise you on this. Many physicians believe that many prescription medications should be discontinued before attempting to conceive. If this is the case, another important variable is the time at which medication should be discontinued before you attempt to conceive.

Besides this, other things that can disrupt any normal pregnancy can still occur. Such pleasures as morning sickness, nausea, and fatigue are still possible. Thrilling, right?

GENETIC CONCERNS

Are you concerned that there may be a possible genetic factor involved in mitral valve prolapse? You may be concerned about passing MVP on to your children. There has been a lot of evidence that mitral valve prolapse is transmitted genetically. So yes, it is possible for children of somebody with MVP to develop MVP as well. This doesn't mean that your children will have the structural defect, or will necessarily develop manifestations of the condition. Remember that there are millions of people who have mitral valve prolapse, and many of them don't experience any noticeable symptoms at all. It is up to each and every person to determine whether or not this is a valid reason to decide against having children. However, these are considerations that you'll want to discuss with your physician. Many people, despite knowing the chances of passing MVP to their children, still plan on (and look forward to) having children.

IF YOU DO CONCEIVE

If you do become pregnant, it is essential to remain in close contact with your doctor. This is especially important for anyone who has a chronic medical condition. This way, if any problems do develop, you'll be able to "nip them in the bud."

Although you may have had an obstetrician before you were diagnosed with mitral valve prolapse, be sure that he or she will take care of you now, knowing that you have MVP. Some doctors may suggest that you switch to a different obstetrician. Is this wrong? You may not be happy about it, but you certainly want to know if a physician feels uncomfortable.

If you can, it's usually a good idea to avoid most medication during pregnancy. But this is not always possible. Aspirin, for example, has been used by many women during their pregnancies, without any damage to the fetus. There are other medications that shouldn't even be considered during pregnancy. Make sure you work closely with your doctor so you know what to use and what not to use.

WHAT ABOUT THE BABY?

If you do have children, you'll want to avoid worrying about whether or not your child is going to develop the condition. Not only will this drive you crazy, but it can frighten your child if apprehension about a diagnosis exists in your home. If MVP eventually is diagnosed, it will be dealt with then. Until such time as the diagnosis occurs, the best way to deal with this is to teach the child proper and appropriate ways of taking care of his or her health through nutrition, exercise, and lifestyle control.

If you have MVP, you may want to have your child checked as part of the normal pediatric physical examination. If the click or murmur of MVP is noticed when the pediatrician listens through a stethoscope, you'll want to gradually implement some of the simpler treatment techniques in order to maintain your child's health as comfortably as possible. Other treatment considerations, such as antibiotics for dental work or other surgical procedures, may be used as required by your child's doctor. However, everything should be done in a very calm, matter-of-fact way, without bringing undue concern to the attention of the child.

ARE YOU PACIFIED?

For your peace of mind, you'll want to answer any question marks that exist about becoming pregnant. The best thing to do is to bring all issues out into the open and discuss them husband and wife, doctor and family. Remember: In most cases, pregnancy should not be a problem at all, especially if your mitral valve prolapse is mild. What's the key to a successful pregnancy? Awareness, supervision, and careful planning. Take all these factors into consideration, and then—good luck!

PART V
Living With Someone With Mitral Valve Prolapse

30

Living With
Someone With MVP—
An Introduction

Illness can create changes in relationships. No kidding! If you live with someone who has MVP, you may have a number of concerns. You may now see that person differently. Maybe you are reminded of your own vulnerability. Maybe you were dependent on that person before; now you have to shoulder more of the burden.

What does all this mean? Although you share the concerns of the individual who has MVP, you also worry about yourself. If you have difficulty dealing with your loved one because of MVP, you're not alone. Often, a medical problem in a loved one will give you a lot of ambivalent feelings. Concerns about the future, your loved one's health, and money may be troublesome to you. This is not unusual.

What if you feel anger toward this person, not because of anything that was done, but because MVP has created changes? This is normal, but may still produce guilt. Why? Because this anger is directed toward somebody who, at the present time, is vulnerable and unable to defend himself or herself. (By the way, throughout this book I have purposely avoided calling the person with MVP a "patient," simply because I believe in emphasizing the person rather than the condition. However, for the sake of convenience and because repeating "your loved one" can become tedious, in this chapter I will refer to the person with MVP as the patient.)

WHAT CAN YOU DO?

If you are close to someone with MVP, you have an important job on your hands. This job is made up of many components, the most important of which is the need to be understanding and supportive. This is very important, whether you live in the same house as the patient or are simply a relative or friend. Remember: People with mitral valve prolapse do not have it easy, but they'll have a much harder time if they feel alone and isolated.

LOYAL LEARNING

A great way for you to help is by learning as much as you possibly can about mitral valve prolapse and its treatment. Do you enjoy worrying? You may have unnecessary worries if you don't know things about the MVP condition that the patient does know. By understanding the patient's condition, you can better provide support and understanding. The knowledge you gain may also be reassuring, especially if you've been "fearing the worst" because you weren't aware of the positive prognosis for most people with MVP.

ENCOURAGE, DON'T PESTER

Encourage adherence to proper management routines or medication needs. But don't badger. If the patient is not taking proper care of himself or herself, there is a limit as to how much you can do to change things. Screaming usually doesn't help (and it can hurt your vocal cords!).

Should you tell the physician if the patient is not taking care of himself or herself? That's a hard question to answer. You don't want to overstep your bounds and be resented. At the same time, you don't want to sit back and let the patient create unnecessary problems. This is especially true if the patient doesn't seem to care. What should you do if the patient just "gives up"? Play each situation by ear. In deciding whether or not to say anything, you should discuss it first with the patient. Voice your concerns, and mention that you're afraid of a problem becoming worse. Listen to the responses before deciding whether to carry it any further.

SYMPATHY?

Because of the difficulties of living with MVP and its treatment, you may sympathize with the patient. You may feel sad about what he or she has to go through. This may help you to provide beneficial support. But don't pity the patient. This can be destructive.

There will be times when the patient is so fatigued that little or nothing can be done. At such times, it is not appropriate for you to insist that the person "get up and do something." That won't make him or her feel better! Try to help out. Try to reduce the patient's pressures at that time. See if you can take over any of his or her obligations or responsibilities; this will certainly make things easier.

At the same time, don't allow the patient to baby himself or herself. In general, if the patient can do something (even if it takes time), let the person do it. If you feel that the patient is "copping out" or malingering, this is something you should both discuss. Try to make life as normal as possible for the patient.

LOYAL FOLLOWING, OR LETTING GO

Don't stay on top of the patient. Sure, you'll want to help. But give the patient enough space to regain some control over his or her own life.

How about doctor's visits? If the patient agrees, you may want to go along for the ride. It might be a good idea for four ears rather than two ears to listen when the doctor is explaining MVP, medication, or other aspects of living with the condition. However, if the patient wants to go alone and feels strongly about it, don't force the issue.

DON'T BE EXTREME

Frequently, friends or relatives go from one extreme to the other. What does this mean? When the patient gets tired, you'll help out. But when the person is no longer tired, will you allow him or her to do what is desired? When feeling better and able to do things, the last thing the patient wants is to be told to get into bed and rest. Have faith in your special someone. If the patient really doesn't feel well, he or she will rest. Otherwise, let 'em be!

THE LONG VS. THE SHORT OF IT

If any patient is going through an acute problem, such as major surgery, a specific treatable illness, or a broken bone, it's a lot easier for the friends and relatives to rally around and provide support and understanding, taking over the responsibilities for the patient while rehabilitation and a cure are taking place. More problems occur with a chronic condition. Sure, there is a period of time when lifestyle has to be reorganized and responsibilities change. But once these changes start taking place, feelings and rough spots stabilize. Life goes on.

But it's still harder in a condition such as mitral valve prolapse because the symptoms may be cyclical. There are times when the patient may not be able to do much and the family has to help out. At other times, your loved one will be able to do a lot more and the family will have to readjust to different roles (maybe similar to the way it used to be). These cyclical changes can create major problems. Because there is no definite time when the problem is going to end, you may have a much more difficult time dealing with the patient's changes. "This is going to go on forever," you may think disgustedly.

HOW TO RESPOND

Can you always be sure of the best response to the patient? You may feel that, at certain times, the best way to respond is with sympathy and understanding. There may be times when you want to joke about MVP. At other times, the best thing may be just to ignore what's going on and walk away. But there's no way for you to know for sure. You can't predict the needs of the patient.

How to help? Lay ground rules. Hopefully, the patient will initiate this. If not, maybe you can start the discussion. Mention your concerns. Talk about your interest in being as supportive as you possibly can, and ask what you can do to help. Things will move more smoothly if you have a good idea of what to do and when to do it. Even if there are no clear-cut, definite answers, at least there will be some constructive communication. You'll be better able to handle future problems.

KEEP TALKING

It is very important to have open lines of communication between you and the patient. This is the only way you can really hear how he or she feels, both physically and emotionally. In this way, you can truly be of help. This doesn't mean that the conversations will always be pleasant. Talking about problems, depression, fears, or pain isn't very enjoyable, especially if you don't have any answers. But with good communication, any difficulties will be overshadowed by the feeling of closeness resulting from shared feelings and concerns.

31

The Child With
Mitral Valve Prolapse

Any time a child is diagnosed with MVP, it is very likely that the doctor doing the diagnosis will immediately have two or three new patients: the child, and the child's mother and/or father. This may be only the tip of the iceberg. The diagnosis of a child with any medical problem can have a devastating effect on the child's family.

It's important for all family members to work through any emotional difficulties they may experience as a result of a child's having mitral valve prolapse. This will keep the family intact and will help the child to better cope with his or her condition. Who else is involved? Friends, teachers, other relatives—all can be affected.

THE CHILD'S PARENTS

The parents of a child diagnosed with MVP probably will experience a whole range of emotional reactions. Feelings of guilt and intense anguish are not uncommon. Parents may regret having genetically transmitted the problem to their child. "Isn't there anything we could have done to prevent this?" they may ask. All these thoughts can be destructive unless they are worked through. Parents should not communicate these feelings to the child, nor should parents make the child feel ashamed.

Watching your child experience any symptoms of MVP can be horrible. It also may be hard for you to make sure that your child takes any necessary medication and gets enough rest.

HOW TO TREAT THE CHILD

You don't want to make things harder for the child with mitral valve prolapse. So don't behave any differently from the way you always did. Don't be more harsh and disciplining, or more lax and indulgent. If you would really rather help the child adjust, then treat the child as a child, not as an unfortunate youngster with a medical problem. Avoid changes in the way you raise your child.

Try not to show painful or unhappy reactions to the child. Imagine how the child will feel seeing unhappiness in loved ones. You can be sure the child will feel guilty. This will only make things worse.

Brothers and sisters at home also can be affected. The degree to which siblings are affected varies, however. This depends on how much extra attention the child with MVP receives, and how brothers and sisters react to this extra attention. Do the other siblings feel like they're losing time with you or other relatives? They may feel that they're being "pushed aside" because of their sibling's condition. This can cause tension between the child with mitral valve prolapse and your other children. Brothers and sisters may become resentful of the extra attention given to the child with MVP. They may not believe that mitral valve prolapse is such a big deal, but believe instead that it is being blown out of proportion for extra attention. On the other hand, the child with MVP may not even want all this attention. This can create guilt!

Emphasize the child rather than the condition. It is better to think of or talk about your child as still a child—a child who happens to have mitral valve prolapse. In addition, try to maintain a calm, emotionally-stable home. This is crucial in keeping the family together. It is harder to change the behavior of more distant family members. How can you keep telling friends and relatives not to bring gifts or shower extra attention on your "poor child"?

As we've said before, parents (as well as others who are close to the child) should learn as much as possible about mitral valve prolapse. The more knowledge you have, the more understanding you can be. You can then be more supportive of your child.

THE CHILD CAN HELP HIMSELF OR HERSELF, TOO

Managing your child's condition should be done matter-of-factly. Make it a regular part of life. It's usually not a good idea to give rewards to your child just for following normal treatment routines. You want the child to learn proper self-care habits, not to expect a reward. But proper self-care will be rewarded, because children who do take good care of themselves will usually feel better.

Regular family habits should continue as before. You all have to learn to live with any restrictions that mitral valve prolapse may impose. Hopefully, everyone in the family, especially the child with MVP, will feel at ease with your child's physician. In that way, any questions or concerns can be dealt with. Your child, especially if very young, will be less able to understand the facts about mitral valve prolapse. But as the child grows, more questions may be asked. You want your child to be able to ask questions, even if you can't provide all of the answers.

HOW DO CHILDREN COPE?

An important factor in determining how well a child will adjust to mitral valve prolapse and its treatment is how well the child handled stress before the onset of the condition. (Does this sound familiar? Of course. This also helps you to understand how adults adjust!) But having MVP may be difficult for a child, especially if physical restrictions interfere with normal activities. You'll want to do everything you can to help the child deal with this. Other problems that may occur for adults also can plague children, such as feelings of isolation, pain, and any side effects from medication.

So what do children do? Some withdraw, sleeping as much as they can, staying away from friends (and even family), and trying not to think about MVP. Others may be much more open about their condition. You can certainly recognize this as a sign of unhappiness. They may even flaunt it, trying to get extra attention. But most children with mitral valve prolapse fall somewhere between these two extremes. Coping strategies can help virtually any child to deal better with MVP.

Some children can be encouraged to learn other enjoyable activities. Swimming is a great sport, and may be good for your child's body. If your doctor approves, why not encourage that? Non-physical activities, such as chess or arts and crafts, can be good outlets. And, of course, doing well academically and developing good reading skills can be a great boost psychologically.

Children Deny, Too!

Children may try to deny some aspects of having mitral valve prolapse. They may fight fatigue, trying to do everything they used to. Or, if they're on medication, they may try to "forget" that. So children may deny that they have a problem. But if they push it away, does that mean it doesn't exist?

You want your child to do what's best. But there are times when children may be able to do more than you think they can. In many cases, children are less sensitive to pain and other negative aspects of MVP than adults. Often, you may be more concerned about the condition than your child is! Try not to be overprotective. However, you should still protect your child. Even when your child pushes too hard, try to allow the child to learn for himself or herself what can and cannot be done. In order to mature while having mitral valve prolapse, the child must be aware, firsthand, of any limitations that may exist.

"Lashing Out"

Rebellion against authority is a normal part of a child's development. When it happens, be sure that you are prepared to deal with it. At the same time, be assured that a child with mitral valve prolapse probably will not seriously hurt himself or herself with tantrum behavior. So deal with rebellion the same way you would if your child didn't have MVP. Ignore it, wait until the child has calmed down, and then talk to your child. Do try to minimize any physical effects of these outbursts. Try to keep the home environment emotionally calm, stable, supportive, and loving.

32

The Adolescent With Mitral Valve Prolapse

Ah, the joys of adolescence! Adolescence can be one of the most difficult periods in one's life. Adolescents are swingers, not because they have such active social lives (although they may), but because their behavior and moods may swing so extremely, from the childish dependence of years gone by to the mature independence of adult years approaching.

Adolescents are frequently insecure and unstable. The adolescent years tend to be sensitive ones. Resentment and rebellion may arise when needs or desires are thwarted. Closeness is also possible on those occasions when adult understanding is shown. The adolescent usually works hard to become more independent, and asserts his or her independence in front of parents. Adolescents want to be on their own. They want to be able to stand up for themselves. At the same time, they don't want to be too different. Mitral valve prolapse and its treatment, can, in many cases, make them feel very different. This can create problems.

For young children, any reductions in activities imposed by either MVP or its treatment may be unpleasant but tolerable. However, for adolescents living in their "glory days," these restrictions may be much more upsetting and depressing.

REBEL TIME

Finding out that an adolescent has MVP can cause major problems. The natural tendency of any parent is to become overprotective when a child has a medical problem. Adolescents almost always object to interference from parents. Why? Because the adolescent wants to become more independent. The fact that parents frequently have difficulty dealing with any medical condition in their adolescent will, in all likelihood, increase adolescent rebellion. Rebellion is a normal part of adolescence, regardless of whether or not mitral valve prolapse is involved. Parents should try not to be overprotective, but as tolerant and understanding as possible. In cases where the adolescent does something wrong, supportive discussions are more appropriate than put-downs and reproaches.

Rebellion may occasionally lead to more physical problems for the adolescent. Why? Because a rebellious teenager may be less diligent with proper MVP self-care. Maybe the adolescent does not take proper care of himself or herself. The adolescent knows that this can be harmful. So what? Hopefully, he or she will learn (without dangerous consequences) that there are better ways to get through adolescence!

PROBLEMS WITH FRIENDS

Making friends is probably one of the most important activities during the adolescent years. Any restrictions imposed because of MVP can reduce available activities. The adolescent may not be able to spend as much time as desired with friends. It may not be possible to go out as often or keep late hours. It may be necessary to cancel plans at the last minute due to extreme fatigue or any discomfort. The adolescent may have a hard time deciding whether to tell friends, and if so, which ones? There may be concern that this information will hurt friendships, new or old. Parents need to be aware of this so they can try to help. In rare cases, the adolescent might even want teachers to provide short classroom lessons about mitral valve prolapse, what it is, and why it's not something that should cause social problems (after learning themselves, of course!). Hopefully, this will bring about more support and understanding.

Many adolescents are embarrassed that they have mitral valve prolapse. To an adolescent, any medical problem can be a stigma.

Teenagers have to be "okay," or it may cost them friends (so they believe). What about the stigma of MVP? Adolescents are at that stage in their lives when social relationships are most important. They may be less able to get involved in physical activities or go to the gym. They may be more reluctant to develop social relationships because of concerns about "feeling different." All this may create a lot of discomfort in their young minds.

It should, therefore, be up to the adolescent to decide whom he or she wants to tell. Teachers probably should know about the illness, since the adolescent may have certain needs or concerns that require more delicate attention. Why might the adolescent choose not to share this information with all friends? He or she might sense that, in some cases, friends would be afraid, upset, or even hostile. Some friends might ignore the adolescent, not wanting to be near someone with a chronic medical problem like mitral valve prolapse. In many cases, unless the condition is revealed, other people may not even know. So let your adolescent make the decision.

If the adolescent seems to be having too much difficulty coping with mitral valve prolapse, professional counseling may be helpful. Sometimes, an objective and supportive person can quickly help a troubled adolescent adjust to an otherwise emotionally-upsetting condition.

WHO HANDLES IT BETTER?

Many adolescents with MVP cope better than their parents do! Parents may feel guilty. Because MVP has its hereditary component, they may feel that they could have done something to prevent it.

Parents frequently feel that it is their responsibility to protect their child from harm, injury, or medical problems. Remember: The adolescent who only feels some occasional chest pain (and adolescents are able to handle pain more effectively than other age groups) and fatigue (which adolescents will either rest through or push past), can usually maintain a fairly normal, active life, despite mitral valve prolapse.

Occasionally, an adolescent may act differently with friends (and in school) than with parents or other family members. Could it be that the adolescent enjoys the protection and concern of parents? Maybe the adolescent puts on a different "face" with family than with friends. Isn't that frequently the case, even if MVP isn't involved? Adolescents may be more willing to confide in their parents than in friends. They don't want friends to think they complain all the time.

Some parents try to protect their adolescents by not telling them everything about their conditions. This is usually not the best approach. Adolescents should know the truth so they can take responsibility for their own management. Adjusting to mitral valve prolapse may take a while. By restricting information, it may take even longer. Anger and bitterness between adolescents and their parents may seriously hurt the relationship.

QUESTIONING THE FUTURE

As the adolescent gets older, certain troublesome questions may come to mind. The adolescent may wonder, "Will someone want to marry me? Will I be able to (or want to) have children? Will I be able to perform my job well enough to keep it? Will I be able to make and keep friends? Will I be able to finish my education? Will I be able to function as a normal member of society?" These questions bother almost all adolescents. Having mitral valve prolapse just makes them more worrisome. The answers? As long as MVP is taken into consideration and lifestyle is adjusted where necessary, the adolescent with mitral valve prolapse should be in the same position to answer these questions as any other healthy teenager.

On to the Future

Well, you've just about finished this book. We've covered a lot of information about MVP. Ongoing research continues to test new medical techniques and medications for treating the condition, as well as further improve the quality of life for the person with MVP.

Perhaps by the time you read this, some drug or treatment may have proven itself to be even more successful than ones currently available. It remains to be seen which new developments can improve your life with MVP. But at least people are working on the problem. It's nice to know that research continues to investigate ways of improving the effectiveness of treatment.

Although it would be impossible to include every possible problem that might be caused by having mitral valve prolapse, I hope that what you've read will help you to develop your own strategies for coping. Because things change, and something that troubles you one day may not trouble you the next (and vice versa), you should use this book as a resource. Whenever you have questions about coping with a certain aspect of MVP, consult these pages. If you have any comments, information you feel is important, or additional questions, feel free to write to me in care of the publisher. I'd be happy to hear from you.

Until such time as there no longer is a medical condition called mitral valve prolapse, keep coping the best you can. Remember, you can always improve the quality of your life, regardless of any medical problem that may come your way.

But for now, look brightly ahead, act proudly, and enjoy life as best you can. I wish all my readers the very best of health and happiness!

Appendix

For Further Reading

Lazarus, A. *In the Mind's Eye.* New York: Rawson Associates Publishers, 1977.

For Further Information

American Heart Association
7320 Greenville Avenue
Dallas, Texas 75231
(214) 373-6300

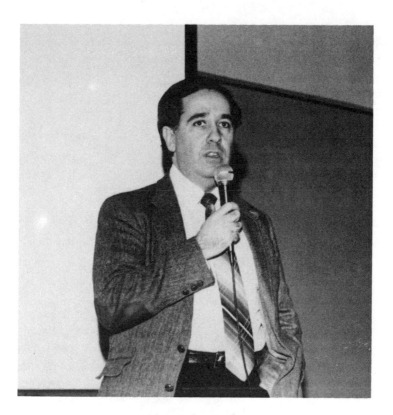

About the Author

Robert H. Phillips, Ph.D., is a practicing psychologist on Long Island, New York. He is the founder and director of the Center for Coping With Chronic Conditions, a multi-service organization helping individuals with chronic illness, and their families. He is involved with a number of local and national medical organizations. In addition, he is the psychologist for and director of the "Cope" program for the Long Island chapter of the Lupus Foundation of America, and is the associate director of the International Coma Recovery Institute.

The author of numerous articles on a variety of subjects in psychology, Dr. Phillips has lectured at conventions, universities, and professional meetings throughout the country, and has appeared on local and national radio and television programs.

Index

Activities of daily living, 188-189
Adolescents with MVP, 257-260
American Heart Association, 195
Amino oxidase inhibitors. *See* MAO inhibitors.
Amoxicillin, 174
Anger, 85-99
    causes of, 86-87
    cognitive techniques for treating, 93-96
    coping with, 91-99
    definition of, 85
    effects on your body, 87-88
    effects on your mind, 88
    good vs. bad, 90-91
    physical techniques for treating, 98
    reactions to, 88-90
    types of, 85-86
Angiogram, 24-25
Antibiotic prophylaxis, 174-175
Anxiety, 135
Anxiety neurosis, 18
Aorta, 4
Arrhythmia, 140, 171
Atrial fibrillation, 15
Atrium, 4, 5

Auscultatory findings, 24
Autonomic nervous system, 12, 15-18, 29, 81, 83, 168, 174, 222, 236
    role of, 16

Bacterial endocarditis, 20-21, 167
Barlow's syndrome, 3, 19
Behavior therapy, 83
Benzodiazapines, 83, 172-173
Beta blockers, 167-168, 171-172
Billow, 3, 9, 15, 23
Blood
    path of, 4-5
Blood regurgitation, 7-8, 9, 12, 15, 21, 23, 130, 167, 174
    progressive, 21
Blood volume, 154, 241-242
Boredom, 119-121
Breath, shortness of, 135, 136, 141-142

Caffeine, 152-153
Calcium channel blockers, 172
Cardiologist, 221
Cardizem, 172
Causes, 11-12